Birthing Your Baby

The Second Stage

Nadine Pilley Edwards
Beverley A. Lawrence Beech

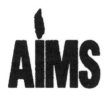

AiMS

ASSOCIATION FOR IMPROVEMENTS IN THE MATERNITY SERVICES

Acknowledgements

We would like to acknowledge the generous contributions of Briony Addis-Jones, Alice Charlwood, Mary Cronk, Mandy Hawke, Louise Hulton, Elizabeth Key, Mavis Kirkham, Jane Munro, Avril Nicholl, Helen Stapleton, Sally Stockley, Pat Thomas, Brenda van der Kooy, Lesley Page, Helen Shallow and Sarah Wickham who have given time to answer our questions read drafts of this booklet. Thanks also to Jean Sutton who generously allowed us to quote from her work and reproduce her drawing of "the pipe", and to Leslie Batchelor for providing the illustrations for this booklet. In addition we would like to thank all the women who shared their birth experiences and knowledge. Their support made this publication possible.

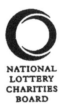

**NATIONAL
LOTTERY
CHARITIES
BOARD**

Supported by the National Lottery Charities Board
Published by AIMS on behalf of the British Maternity Trust
©AIMS March 2001
ISBN 1 874413 12 6

Contents

Preface

This booklet is for those who would like to know more about the second stage of labour, although in this size booklet it is not possible to cover every aspect. For example, we do not include specific information for women who plan to decide during labour to have an epidural. Nor do we give specific information for those women expecting twins, or for women whose babies are breech at term – though the information may still be of use to them.»

There are many variations to the "textbook" birth which nevertheless can be regarded as normal. It is often said that "no two labours are the same". Many women find that each of their labours can be very different.

In essence this booklet discusses two different approaches to the second stage of labour: physiological and actively managed. There are ongoing discussions about the benefits and drawbacks of encouraging a woman to

---

» Having twins, or a breech baby need not essentially be different from having a baby whose head is the presenting part, though it is essential, in the absence of complications, that women planning to have twins or breech babies vaginally are encouraged to follow the rhythms of their own bodies throughout labour. This midwifery approach to a breech or twin birth supports the physiological process and if it becomes apparent that the woman is going to need help, a caesarean section is usually recommended. The use of oxytocic drugs and continuous electronic fetal monitoring during a normal birth which constrains the woman is not recommended. For further information on these topics, see AIMS 1998, Banks 1998, Cronk 1998a; Cronk 1998b; Evans 1997; Cronk 2000.

find her own way of birthing her baby compared with directing her behaviour during the second stage of labour. This booklet considers the issues surrounding each approach.

It is, of course, in the privileged context of a relatively affluent and healthy society that this booklet is written. Most women can indeed look forward to having a live, healthy baby. However, babies are born to many different women in many different circumstances. Women have their own individual needs during pregnancy, birth and the period after birth and this booklet is, of course, limited by its cultural context. The second stage of labour may be defined, described and experienced differently by women of this and other cultures and their needs may be different from those suggested here.

For many women labour cannot easily be broken down into stages. Because this booklet primarily concerns the second stage we have focused on this but at the same time have attempted to provide a context which recognises the process as a whole and the wide range of different experiences women can have. We have done this by describing how labour progresses and how women move into the second stage of labour; what happens during the second stage from transition to birth and the physiological approach to the second stage. We have then considered the medicalisation of birth in an historical context and described active management of labour and possible complications. Finally, we have looked at the way in which birth plans and labour companions can help the woman.

We have attempted to set out some of the views, debates, research and experiences concerning the second stage of labour as clearly as possible, but inevitably these can be conflicting and confusing. We have also covered issues which relate to the second stage of labour – even though this may not be immediately apparent. Some of these topics are subjects of wide debate themselves. We have therefore attempted to cover the most salient points and refer readers to other articles and books for further discussion.

Introduction

When we try to answer women's questions, and support them, we are using a combination of information from many sources. The bedrock of our knowledge is what we have learned from many other women's stories of pregnancy and birth, good and bad, over the years – and often those of their partners as well. Each woman asking for help joins the circle, and becomes a giver, as well as a receiver. Woven into our text is the invaluable information we get from midwives – anecdotes, experience and often their cries for help. Some obstetricians and GPs, and even medical students, provide yet more data. Then there is the solid, frequent exchange of ideas and information with other organisations – especially the National Childbirth Trust. Are they seeing more of the latest problem we are getting?

All this is backed up by our struggle to keep up with the latest research, so that we are as well informed and up-to-date as we can be. Although we read, and often quote, research data, we always look at it from the perspective of our callers. Does it make sense and ring true, is it even relevant, in the light of what mothers teach us?

"*If only I had known*", "*If only I had insisted*", "*If only I had refused*" are phrases we commonly hear after births have gone wrong – physically or emotionally or both. Trying to give birth is too often a clash between what the woman's body and spirit are telling her, and the pattern of care she receives.

The instructions she is receiving from professionals can stifle, or reduce her confidence in, her inner voice. The first birth can be particularly important, because that is when she has to learn that it is there, and to listen and heed. Even some "good" births, we find, are not as good as they might have been – though women are reluctant to criticise – because, for example, midwives chattered, however quietly, and broke the spell.

We know when we provide material about birth, it is information which women will often have to use in the most difficult of circumstances – at a time when their mind is operating in a different way on a different level, when they may be in pain and anxious, and when they are surrounded by confident professionals who "know" what is good for them. However much you know, having the skill and the power to use your knowledge in those circumstances is something else again. Women intuitively feel that they have to try to get what they need by not offending or challenging their attendants.

They also tell us how aware they were of the constraints that professionals were working under. Midwives and doctors also have to try to survive the culture of the institutions which educate and employ them. *"The holders of power, predominantly males, will be invisible; their authority will be present but they will be out of sight. The design of the labour ward...is evidence of this invisibility of power"* (Hunt and Symonds, 1995). Above all there are the constraints on time. Nature's time, baby's time, birthing time vary, but the set pattern of what is considered "normal" or "safe" in the hospital does not. Too often there is a mismatch, which either leads to unnecessary intervention, or subterfuge by a supportive midwife to "allow" the mother to follow the needs of her own body.

Of course we know that separating out the second stage – or any stage – is artificial. This booklet is just a way of helping readers (and ourselves) to focus on manageable quantity of information, but also to focus on certain issues.

Part of our work is to deal with the misinformation women have already acquired from the media. Hardly a week goes by without our seeing on the television a birth scene where husbands, midwives, doctors, ambulancemen, are exhorting labouring women to "push! push! push!" The fact that the rugby-coach approach does not help, and is even damaging is unknown to most of the population.

Women also tell us of their loss of pushing ability after over-stimulation with oxytocin drips, or their frustration at lost or muted pushing ability with epidurals. Others recognise after the event that their difficulty in getting the baby out was related to their lack of privacy, or the attitudes and behaviour of those around them.

I was always impressed by the Canadian randomised trial of Leboyer childbirth (where babies after delivery are cared for in a quiet, darkened, gentle atmosphere) which showed that the Leboyer mothers had significantly shorter labours. Why should the mere knowledge that your baby will be treated in such a way make labour faster? Or perhaps we should realise that the bright lights, noise, lack of privacy are causing labour to be longer (Nelson et al, 1980).

Whether or not the woman can freely adopt the position that feels right for birthing is a useful way of judging the quality of care for normal birth. We believe that every hospital should provide annual statistics on positions in which women gave birth – and those which do not show variety, or which exclude all fours, should be examining their practice.

When I attended a meeting at the Royal College of Obstetricians and Gynaecologists on postnatal incontinence, I asked the obstetricians, physiotherapists and midwives present what contribution positions used for labour and delivery made to the risk. Answers came there none. It was clearly a question many of them had not thought about.

One of the most important consumer themes is time – and how much time the woman is "allowed" for the second stage – or any other part of birth. Labour, birthing and placenta expulsion should be in the woman's body and spirit time, the baby's time, just the time it takes for this woman, this baby to be birthed – unless there is good cause to intervene. The apparent gaps when doctors (and some midwives) think "nothing" is happening so they have to do something are often a precious and essential part of the process. That is why I particularly valued the description of midwife Mary Cronk's "rest and be thankful" time, in this book.

Again, for water birth, even hospitals which actually "allow" women to labour in the pool they advertise as part of their amenities, may insist women leave it before the baby comes. One of our contacts was severely traumatised by the sudden escalation of pain after she left the water, particularly as – not surprisingly – there was a much longer delay before the birth than midwives had expected.

Nadine Edwards, AIMS' Vice Chair, is a birth teacher and has often acted as birth companion. She is also a gifted researcher. Beverley Beech, our main helpline contact, is in touch with women every day. This booklet is based on published research. But the authors who have read and quoted it, to distil information for women, were in a position to assess its truth and relevance from long experience of working within AIMS. By sharing our information with our readers, our aim is to provide some basic knowledge which will help them to develop confidence in themselves and their own reactions.

Jean Robinson
Hon. Research Officer
AIMS

Getting to the Second Stage of Labour

"As a human female physiologic process, labour is both a universal phenomenon and a highly individual experience. It is predictable that it will occur, but unpredictable and idiosyncratic in its actual occurrence. Despite attempts to package labour into discrete phases and stages, it is better understood as a whole, with an ebb and flow and rhythms of its own. It is intensely physical and emotional, consuming all of one's attention and energy, yet life-giving and empowering in that intensity. How then is it possible to manage labour?" (Kaufman, 1993)

During pregnancy many women will have estimated the date their babies are due themselves, or they will have been given an estimated date by their midwife or obstetrician. Most babies arrive sometime between 37 and 42 weeks. In the later weeks or days a woman's uterus will begin to prepare for labour by having "practice" contractions. These are called Braxton Hicks contractions and they can sometimes give the woman the impression that she is in labour.

These contractions may occur for a few hours, or more, in the days before labour starts. The first contractions may be like period pains and early on women may be uncertain whether or not they are in labour. As time passes the contractions become more powerful so that the woman will find that she has to stop what she is doing and focus on relaxing.

Although each woman's labour is unique, in established labour her contractions usually become regular and increase in intensity and frequency, but labour is not generally considered to be established until her contractions are regular, strong and dilating her cervix.

Typically in midwifery text books the second stage of labour is described as beginning when the woman's cervix is fully open and she is ready to give birth to her baby (see Morrin, 1997; and see Sleep, 1993). As the woman's cervix becomes fully dilated, she may experience what is referred to as 'transition'. Midwives attending a woman who wants a spontaneous approach to the second stage of labour usually give fewer instructions.

When the mother shows signs of bearing down she is neither encouraged to push or not to push, but to follow what her body needs to do.» She may stay in upright or kneeling positions, or may move into a more upright position instinctively. The atmosphere is usually quieter and calmer, with the focus on the woman and maintaining her comfort as far as possible. The midwife may give feedback and encouragement that all is as it should be.

» Unfortunately it can be difficult for a woman to follow her instincts, particularly if she finds herself in clinical surroundings, attended by people she has not seen before, interrupted by people entering the room. If she feels out of touch with her own body or is unaccustomed to making decisions for herself, being encouraged to follow her body's instincts can feel almost impossible. However, childbirth is a rite of passage and when a woman has been encouraged and supported, her confidence can be enormously enhanced. Or, conversely, when she does not have support and encouragement her confidence can be seriously diminished.

Ferguson's Reflex

This term describes the release of natural oxytocin (a hormone that makes the uterus contract) in the woman's body during labour and birth. It occurs in different ways at different stages of labour and birth and is responsible for keeping the whole process going.

For the reflex to work well, the woman's hormonal balance should remain undisturbed. This is why she needs privacy and a calm atmosphere, as this environment enhances oxytocin release (see Odent, 1998; and see Robertson, 1994).

The woman needs to be protected from unnecessary disturbance or interruptions, and free of emotional and psychological anxieties, as far as possible, as these can hinder oxytocin release and affect the frequency and efficiency of her contractions. Any interventions, such as the use of syntocinon or epidurals, tend to inhibit this reflex. The unfamiliar hospital environment can have the same effect on some women.

During the second stage the pressure of the baby's head on the woman's pelvic floor muscles, the distension of her vagina and the stretching of her perineum, triggers the release of oxytocin. There is a further surge of natural oxytocin at the moment of crowning, which assists in the birth of the placenta and protects the woman from excessive bleeding after birth (see Further Reading – Edwards, 1999).

What Happens During the Second Stage

"Entering the second stage of labour can be an almost overwhelming experience for a labouring woman. Some find it liberating and exciting – at last the end of labour is coming, they can push, something is happening; for others it is the hardest part of labour, when they can become demoralised, feeling they can't go on, even believing they are going to die".

(McCandlish, 1997)

Transition

The second stage of labour is often preceded by a series of tumultuous contractions – often women experience these as long, powerful and painful. These bring about the complete dilation of her cervix. This can be accompanied by shaking, nausea or vomiting, and feelings of confusion, despair, or panic. Women can become irritable or angry for a time.

Often women will feel:

"I can't do this any more".

"I want a caesarean section NOW".

"I can't do this, it's stuck".

Your Baby's Position

It might be helpful later in your pregnancy to find out how your baby is lying. Although this has not been researched, if your baby is in an occipito posterior (OP) presentation – where your baby's back lies close to your own back (see page 66) – you can adopt certain positions and make minor changes in your lifestyle to try to encourage your baby into a favourable position before labour starts. Of course, there are some babies who, despite all efforts, for whatever reason stay posterior.

Before labour begins, particularly during the last six weeks of your pregnancy you can adopt more upright, forward leaning postures by:

- Avoiding bucket seats in cars and, if possible, long car journeys.
- Avoiding reclining in easy chairs or settees with your feet up – which women are often encouraged to do during pregnancy – or sitting with your knees higher than your hips.
- Sitting in upright chairs or leaning forward over some cushions. If you wish to recline lie on your left side and put a cushion or two under your right knee. Trying not to sit with your legs crossed.
- If the baby is breech or posterior, crawling for 10-20 minutes a day to encourage your baby to turn.
- Going swimming and walking when you can.

Some might make lots of noise, or cry; whilst others become very silent, concentrated, and uncommunicative. Because these last dilating contractions can be so intense, this is often a time when women who had been coping without much pain relief, will want to give up and go home.

"I said 'I want to go home', which is ridiculous
because I was at home"

Some women want an epidural or other analgesia.» By this time, however, the birth is usually imminent, and by the time an epidural takes effect the baby is usually born.

With the calm reassurance, care and understanding of their attendants, they can be helped to work through this phase to give birth to their baby.

Each woman's experience of transition can be very different. The woman may be unsure what to do, not knowing whether she feels like bearing down or not. Once bearing down sensations begin, the contractions often feel more defined, shorter and further apart, less painful and easier to cope with than the overwhelming, dilating contractions at the end of the first stage of labour.

» Epidurals can have a number of adverse affects on progress in the second stage of labour, and the likelihood of needing a caesarean or a forceps delivery will be substantially increased (Thorp and Breedlove, 1996).

The woman may become more aware of her surroundings again – chatting and relaxing between contractions, or she may close her eyes and focus in order to adapt to the new messages her body is sending her, once expulsive contractions become clearly established.

'Rest and Be Thankful'

Alternatively, once the powerful contractions of the first stage have fully opened the woman's cervix, there may be a lull when the contractions die down, or stop for a while.

It may last a while, or be so fleeting as to pass unnoticed. At this point the woman's cervix is fully dilated and begins to draw up and the baby's head slips out of the uterus. It has been suggested that time is needed for the fibres of the uterus to lighten up again around the baby's body and that this may explain why some women experience this lull (Simkin, 1990).

Midwife, Mary Cronk calls this the "rest and be thankful period",» and many practitioners share her view that this is a normal, physiological and beneficial interval which gives both the woman and the baby an opportunity to rest (some women fall asleep if they're left undisturbed), relax, and generally gather strength before expulsive contractions begin.

» The Rest and Be Thankful is a long, steep, mountain road between two lochs in the Trossachs in Scotland, when one reaches the top one can "rest and be thankful".

However, this lull is sometimes interpreted by midwives and doctors as the woman's labour "failing to progress" and instead of resting and being grateful for the break, her waters may be broken, if they have not already done so, and a drip, containing a synthetic hormone, syntocinon, may be set up to start contractions again.

There are anecdotal stories of this lull lasting several hours or women eating a large meal between dilation and giving birth (Armstrong, 1987). However, in hospital there may be policies in place that suggest intervening after a set period of time (see pages 46 and 58). Any woman who is told at this time that she is failing to progress and that her waters should be broken or a drip set up, or both, might like to consider how she feels, and ask those caring for her if there are any problems with the baby.

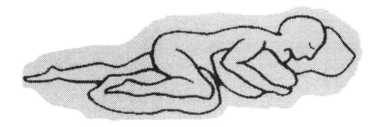

If both woman and baby are fine the woman may decide to wait to see if the labour progresses without intervention. She could use the lull to rest and perhaps catnap, or even sleep. Some like to have a drink or freshen up and have a wash. The passage of time alone should not necessitate intervention if the woman and baby are well (see McCandlish, 1997).

Bearing Down

The active phase of the second stage begins when the woman's uterus begins to contract strongly and she feels a strong urge to bear down during contractions. Ideally, at the onset of the second stage of labour the baby's head will be well flexed i.e. with its chin tucked in. As downward pressure is exerted on the baby by the woman's contracting uterus, typically its head tucks well in under the curve of her spine (see Sutton and Scott, 1995) as it negotiates the soft tissues and bony structure of the pelvis in a series of small movements.

As labour advances the baby usually turns and moves slightly to take advantage of the widest available space in the woman's pelvis as it descends. When it meets the resistance of the woman's pelvic floor it begins to rotate.»

The contractions can be felt by placing a hand on the woman's abdomen – her uterus seems to tighten, even knot (see Simkin, 1990). If encouraged to follow her instincts the woman will usually bear down briefly, breathe quickly, hold her breath briefly and grunt and strain during the surges (Caldeyro Barcia, 1978).

» Rotation and descent of the baby's head may be more difficult with an epidural, as it interferes with the bearing down reflex. The reduced tone in the abdominal muscles can make it more difficult for the woman to push (Hannington-Kiff, 1993). In addition, loss of tone in the pelvic floor (motor blockade) can weaken the pelvic floor musculature and interfere with the progression of the baby's head, preventing natural rotation.

Constance Beynon (1957), observed slight straining until the baby's head begins to distend the woman's pelvic floor and the urge to bear down becomes irresistible. Contractions during the second stage of labour also vary in strength. Some are strong, where the baby moves down noticeably, and some are mild where the baby moves very little, if at all.

Interestingly, where pushing is undesirable or impossible, perhaps due to maternal heart problems or paralysis, often labour progresses smoothly and well. In her study, Beynon observed that fewer episiotomies were performed and forceps were used less frequently.

There is evidence that spontaneous bearing down does not have a negative effect upon either the woman or the baby (Paine and Tinker, 1992) and may have benefits. An earlier study (Maresh et al, 1983) showed more spontaneous births when the woman did not bear down until the baby's head was visible at the vulva. In this particular study, second stages were slightly longer but were not harmful to woman or baby.

The woman may need increased support and contact from those around her, as she makes new sounds from the very depths of her being, bends her knees and drops down during contractions as she feels urges to bear down.

"I grunted and made lots of noise."

She may experience pain as the baby's head moves lower. Her waters may break – if her waters have remained intact, this is the most likely time for them to rupture spontaneously (Sforza-Brewer and Green, 1981; Inch, 1989).»

As the baby moves further and further down, the pushing urge becomes irresistible and the woman's abdominal muscles and diaphragm contract involuntarily to help birth her baby. At the same time her rectum is flattened into the sacral curve of her spine. She may pass urine involuntarily as she pushes. If her bladder is empty it is pushed up safely out of the way, which is why the midwife will encourage the woman regularly to empty her bladder during the labour.

At this point, the pressure of the baby's head may make the woman feel the need to defecate and she may feel more comfortable sitting on the toilet for a while. Pressure from the baby's head usually causes any faecal matter to be expelled (although many women will have had diarrhoea in early labour).

*"I didn't want to stop pushing as I could
feel the baby moving back in."*

This is normal and expected by midwives who will clear up and dispose of the small amount of faeces quickly, even if it occurs while the woman is in a pool or bath.

» The woman's waters can break at any stage of very late pregnancy, or during labour without problems, but the midwife may advise a vaginal examination (VE), to ensure that the cord has not descended in front of the baby's head (cord prolapse). This is very unlikely to be the case if the baby's head has engaged and is deep in the woman's pelvis, as there is no room for the baby's cord to slip through. Cord prolapse can also be excluded by checking the baby's heartbeat; if this is normal, a VE may not be necessary.

Often, if the woman is having her first baby, the baby's head moves gradually through her pelvis, moving forwards through the vagina during the contractions, but slipping back again in between contractions.

Birthing Your Baby

The baby's head moves gradually – or sometimes quickly – through the woman's pelvis until the widest presenting part of the baby – usually its head – finally emerges.

"To feel her move through me was amazing."

The woman may require help and encouragement to relax and open rather than tense her pelvic floor, buttocks and thigh muscles during this often difficult active phase. If the woman has not had a baby before, the gradual crowning» of the baby's head enables her vagina to stretch gradually and slowly open for the baby to be born, ideally without causing grazing or tearing.

Crowning may pass very quickly followed by a feeling of immense relief, or may be marked by confusion, pain and intense feelings. As the baby's head crowns, pain is sometimes felt as burning and stretching, like "a ring of fire".

"It's like a Chinese burn on your fanny".

» Crowning is defined as the passage of the widest presenting diameter through the outlet rim of the woman's birth canal.

A Rim of Cervix

The woman may be pushing spontaneously for some time and feel that the baby is not moving down. She and the midwife may decide that a vaginal examination would be helpful to check what is happening and if there is any of her cervix still undilated (often referred to as a rim or lip). This appears to be more common if the membranes have ruptured or have been ruptured.

Although there is little research evidence, it is believed by many midwives and doctors that where a rim of cervix remains, particularly if the woman is having her first baby, it can become swollen if she follows her urge to push – this might inhibit the baby's descent.

In these circumstances, the woman will often be advised by her midwife to resist the urge to bear down. Some women have found that lying on their sides for a while or adopting a "knee-chest" position helps, as it relieves the pressure on the cervix.

Alternatively, getting into a birth pool or a bath or pretending to blow out candles during a contraction helps reduce the urge to bear down. The midwife continues to observe and encourage the woman. If she considers there are problems she may wish to consult a colleague. Some practitioners will attempt to ease the rim of cervix over the baby's head. This may or may not be successful.

However, in one review, it has been suggested that it may be unhelpful to direct a woman at any stage during labour, as it may distance her from her "bodily sensations" making it difficult for her to respond to later urges to bear down (Roberts and Woolley, 1996). Such instructions may also make the woman dependent on her caregivers to tell her what to do.

The reviewers go on to suggest that there may be no detrimental effects from the woman responding spontaneously to her own bodily urges to bear down and that these slight, early, bearing down urges may help dilate the woman's cervix when it is nearly dilated, soft and retracting, and the baby's head is rotating and descending. In fact, up to two-thirds of women may experience an expulsive urge before they reach full cervical dilation (see McCandlish, 1997).

At the time of crowning women are often urged to hold their breath and "push through the pain". However, the burning sensation may be a signal not to push too hard so as to give the woman's perineum the opportunity to stretch slowly, thereby avoiding lacerations, bruising or tears, whereas pushing hard at this stage might actually cause a tear (See Valsalva manoeuvre, page 59).

Having crowned, the baby's head cannot slip back any more and the midwife will usually encourage the woman not to rush. Mary Cronk talks about letting the head slide out. In Britain, when a woman is about to push her baby out, it is common practice for midwives to "guard" the perineum with one hand, hold the baby's head with the other hand and guide and lift it as it emerges, and then lift the baby out by the shoulders. Some midwives will wait and see, and intervene in this way only if there is an indication.»

With the next contraction, the baby's face sweeps over the woman's perineum, draining any liquor from its nose and mouth, usually eliminating the need for the midwife to suction the baby's airways with a mucus extractor. She may suggest the woman pants rather than pushes as the head is born. After the head is born, the baby turns to one side so that the shoulders can slide through sideways one at a time and then, usually, the whole body slithers out more easily in the next contraction.

"I felt burning for a split second and then she was there –
I couldn't believe I'd had a baby."

» In an effort to determine whether or not these practices affect subsequent perineal pain, midwives undertook a large, multi-centre, randomised controlled trial, called the HOOP trial (Hands On – Or Poised), in which each woman who agreed to take part was randomly allocated to a hands on or off approach thereby ensuring a similar group of women to compare (McCandlish, 1998).

The main points are that the differences in perineal pain after the birth were in fact very small between the two groups. It is difficult to know from the trial whether it was indeed the practice of hands on or off the baby's head that affected pain after birth – or whether it could have been another factor – such as position – or other components of care.

Its conclusions raised many questions and highlighted the need to look at the different components of care in relation to each other. In our opinion there is now a need to design a trial which could identify what aspects of care may damage the woman's perineum and cause postnatal pain, without necessarily making assumptions about these beforehand.

Midwife, Jean Sutton claims that the posterior shoulder is always born first but other midwives find that this only happens occasionally, especially if the woman is on all-fours (Cronk 1999, personal communication). A baby in the posterior position occasionally does not rotate and is born face up. Sometimes a baby is born with its hand or arm emerging beside its head.

There may be 1-2 contractions between the birth of the head and the body. If the woman has had a baby before, the second stage is usually shorter and the baby may descend and be born in few contractions.»

Sometimes the baby is born from head to foot in one contraction! The woman may take a moment or two to take in the fact that she has given birth, or may immediately begin to touch or pick up and embrace her baby.

» *Shoulder Dystocia.* In the highly unlikely event of there being a difficulty with the baby's shoulders, the midwife will follow a procedure which has been shown to be effective in freeing them – the McRoberts' Manoeuvre (Coates, 1997). This will probably require you to lie flat on your back and bring your knees as far up as you can (so that they are up towards your ears) and a second person, midwife or doctor, may press quite hard on the lower part of your tummy to help free the baby's shoulder. Or, if you are lying on your back, the midwife will ask you to get onto all fours, or lie on your left side. These procedures need to be done calmly but quickly.

A Physiological Approach to the Second Stage

Imagine that you are a midwife: you are assisting at someone else's birth. Do good without show or fuss. Facilitate what is happening rather than what you think ought to be happening. When the baby is born, the mother will rightly say: "we did it ourselves".
Lao Tzu, The Tao of Leadership (5th Century BC)

Over the centuries there have always been advocates for a gentle approach to birth, with minimum intervention (see Donnison, 1988). More recently, childbirth activists and educators (Balaskas, 1991; Kitzinger, 1987; Simkin, 1990) have questioned the growing medical management of birth.

A greater understanding of the physiology of the second stage of labour, based on more research, is emerging and in some quarters trust in the woman's body has begun to take the place of the fear and urgency which many health professionals felt in the past.

The principles on which a physiological approach is based includes recognition of the fact that the subtle physiological changes, including hormone secretion, which occur in the baby during the second stage improves its ability to adapt to life outside the womb. More doctors' and midwives' views are changing, so that they now regard the well being of the woman and baby as more important than imposing arbitrary time limits, on the birth process. The duration of the second stage in itself, is not necessarily of importance, unless complications arise (Saunders et al, 1992; see also section on 'Time limits' page 58).

As suggested earlier, women instinctively tend to bear down for short periods, using slow or light rapid breathing. There is evidence to suggest that early forceful pushing during the latent phase of the second stage is not only exhausting and demoralising, but slows it down and results in fewer spontaneous births.

As early as 1957 obstetrician Constance Beynon described the beneficial effects of a physiological approach but this work was largely ignored. Nowadays it is more widely accepted that when gradual stretching of the woman's perineum occurs there is less injury to her and less sudden compression and decompression of the baby's skull. If the woman's perineum is allowed to stretch gradually it is usually able to thin and stretch enough to accommodate the baby.

Upright Positions for a Physiological Birth

In most cultures, and in the West until the 18th century, women used semi-squatting, kneeling and standing positions to give birth. The woman usually finds it easier to bear down in this position. She works with gravity, her pelvic diameters are increased, less pushing is necessary (useful for a woman who is tired), the base of her spine is able to move slightly, allowing extra space for the passage of the baby, the woman can relax her pelvic floor muscles more easily, and the baby's head exerts more even pressure as it stretches the woman's perineum and opens her vulva. Womens' bodies are well-designed for giving birth in upright or in an all fours position but not when they are required to lie on their backs routinely, or when they are propped up by pillows. As obstetrician, Professor Roberto Caldeyro Barcia (1985) remarked, "the only position worse than lying on your back for birth is hanging by your heels from a chandelier".

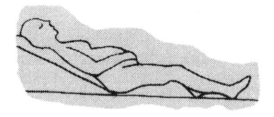

Jean Sutton (Sutton and Scott, 1995) points out that "a woman in an upright position (supported squatting, on a birth stool or kneeling with upper body raised and supported) is in the best physiological posture for a straightforward birth."

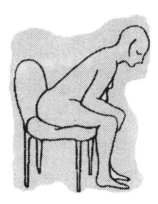

When uninterrupted and encouraged to follow her body's messages the woman is more likely to move into positions which enable her baby to descend and birth. These rarely include lying down or drawing her knees up towards her shoulders. However, there are powerful social influences on positions for the second stage of labour. If not encouraged to change position, women will often stay on a bed, even if they feel very uncomfortable. A review of research findings and anecdotal evidence suggest that the position the woman adopts affects the course of labour and birth.

A systematic Cochrane review (Gupta, 2000) and other studies of women who were upright during labour found that they had shorter labours, less discomfort, less intolerable pain, shorter second stages, fewer tears and fewer episiotomies (de Jong, 1997; NCT, 1993; Roberts and Woolley, 1996). One study showed that mobility shortens the first stage of labour by up to several hours and the strength of contractions have been shown to be affected by position and their efficiency to be almost doubled in upright positions (Mendez-Bauer et al, 1976).

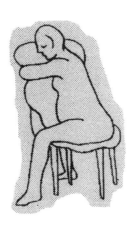

Positions that move the baby's weight so as to avoid compression of the woman's major vein and artery which run between her uterus and her spine will tend to improve blood flow to the baby and reduce the risk of fetal distress.

Being upright, free to move and lean forward in a variety of positions is very helpful, as was borne out by a Japanese study (Nakai, 1998) where pregnant women were, curiously enough, *laid face down* on a bed with a large hole for their abdomens, so that the babies were not squashed. The blood flow to the babies was studied with Doppler ultrasound.

This was compared with babies whose mothers were lying on their left sides, right sides, or backs. The researchers found that when women were face down, compression was completely relieved and the baby got the best possible blood supply. Being on all fours would presumably have shown similar results.

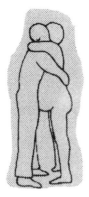 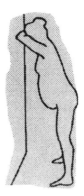

The best position for a woman to adopt is the one she takes up intuitively but it depends upon her being encouraged throughout her labour to follow her instincts. This can be difficult to achieve if the woman is cared for by attendants who tell her what to do, or if she expects to be told what to do.

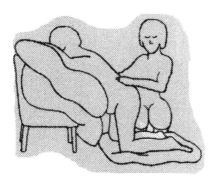

Squatting

In recent years Western (Caucasian) women have been encouraged to squat by some childbirth educators and midwives. It was thought that this would maximise the space in the pelvis and best help the birth process (see Balaskas, 1991) but this is often a difficult position for women who have used stools or chairs since childhood.

Women who are accustomed to squatting in their day-to-day lives squat differently and find it easier to adopt a squatting position for birth than most Caucasian women.

Furthermore, Sutton and Scott (1995) suggests that a full squat where the woman's bottom is close to the floor actually works against the process of birth by preventing her from moving her pelvis in response to the birth ejection reflex: "The best way for a woman to be in a supported squat is to be flat footed, straight-backed with her bottom at least 45cm above the floor. The angle between the spine and the pubic bone is 90 degrees. Squatting in this way allows the woman to "throw" her pelvis forwards as the fetal head extends into the birth canal lifting the sacrum and coccyx out of the way.

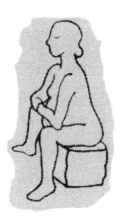

"The woman's hip joints are in front of her ankles when she does this involuntary thrust of her pelvis. She also must have support when squatting in this way, which is best given by her labour support person(s). The woman could also lean forwards, resting her hands on a table or furniture of similar height, with her feet flat, apart, and bend her knees". Studies have shown that when a woman assumes a standing squat position for the birth her pelvic diameter is increased by up to 2cm (Russell, 1982).

Hands and knees ✳ ✳ ✳

When European women are free to adopt whatever position they feel like they will often spend time on their hands and knees during labour and birth. As the baby descends, the woman will often intuitively raise the upper half of her body to help birth her baby. Some women will grip their partners around the neck, grasp the bed head or lean onto something or someone.

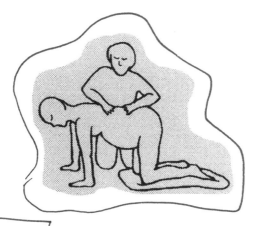

Left-side position

If a woman wants rest and does not feel comfortable upright or on her hands and knees she may find it more comfortable to lie on her left side (called "left lateral" position), rather than on her back. If the woman is tired, lying on her side still allows her pelvis to open for the birth of her baby.

Lying on the left side (or being on hands and knees) may be of particular benefit if the woman has had a previous episiotomy and she and her midwife are working together to avoid damage to her perineum. Some women will move into this position spontaneously and a few women will give birth in semi-recumbent positions. These positions may also help to slow down the birth if the baby is coming very quickly.

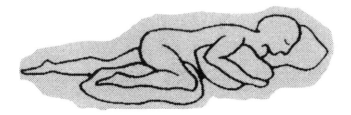

There are many variations to the positions shown in the diagrams. Women and their partners may find it helpful to try them out during pregnancy to see how comfortable they feel and to develop confidence to try different positions.

Emotional Aspects of the Second Stage of Labour

"As well as quietness and calm, the women valued praise, positivity, simplicity, reassurance and gentle encouragement in their midwives to help them get through the second stage. They talked of how important it was that the midwife gave them confidence. Confidence in both the midwife's skills and their own ability to give birth. The midwife needs to believe that the woman can do it and convey that belief to her". (Anderson, 2000)

The birth of a baby can be as emotional, spiritual, sensual or sexual as it is physical. Much depends on how the birth unfolds. It may also depend on how comfortable the woman feels with those around her and the environment in which she gives birth. It may also depend on her own beliefs and expectations. Midwife, Tricia Anderson (2000), in her research on women's experiences of the second stage, suggests that the woman is at her most vulnerable as she approaches birth, and needs to feel completely secure, respected and nurtured in order to finally "let go" and allow herself to give birth. The behaviour of the people around her is crucial in enabling her to feel powerful and able to give birth. **»**

» Given the current pressures on the NHS maternity services it is rare that women or midwives will be in any position to develop trusting relationships. Midwives are rarely enabled to manage their own case loads and look after women thoughout pregnancy, birth and post natally. It is not uncommon for a woman to find she is allocated to a 'team' of 10 or more midwives and will have no idea which of those midwives will be on duty when she goes into labour. Even during labour, the report First Class Delivery (Audit Commission, 1997) revealed that almost 50% of women were attended by 4 or more different midwives during their labours. Without continuity of carer, the trust and support a woman might need is unable to develop and she may not feel safe enough during the birth (Anderson, 2000; Edwards, 2000). At present only independent midwives and a few NHS midwives are able to offer this kind of care.

The actual moments of birth are both an intense completion and transition for woman and baby.

"It was hard work but very satisfying."

A woman may be brimming over with a variety of intense emotions, from exhaustion or relief, to a feeling of fulfilment and joy.

"I felt like a sort of overpowering energy".

Anthropologist, Sheila Kitzinger (1985) observed that breathing during the second stage of labour often resembles that during sexual excitement and orgasm. There is a rhythmic building of tension, until the point of greatest stretching and then a sudden release, as the baby slips out of the woman's body.

Giving birth is often seen as divorced from sexuality, despite the baby being the culmination of a sexual act. In a stark hospital setting with too little privacy and in the presence of strangers, this is perhaps not surprising. It may also reflect the discomfort of those present. Despite this, some women do experience birth as an intensely sensual, even orgasmic event.

"As much as I was in severe pain and giving birth to a baby it was really quite a sexual experience, how can pushing a baby out be sexual? Maybe sensual would be a better word".

"The actual giving birth is slightly orgasmic, there's something
so sensual about having a baby".

Qualitative research and women's and midwives' experiences show us just how deeply giving birth can affect a woman's sexuality and how it can also be seriously affected by past traumas. For some women these past traumas can inhibit giving birth. As one midwife described:

"One of the longer and more intense pushing phases I helped with lasted more than five hours. The mother was young, athletic and strong, yet each push yielded the tiniest progress. A lot of things were happening during this time. She was testing and gaining reassurance from her mate that his devotion was sincere and could endure difficult times. She was showing her sisterly/motherly/housemate/friend that she was not a child anymore. She was breaking through her reluctance to stand up for herself and ask to have her wants and needs met. These things I could see. I did not know, nor did she, that she was also completing internal recovery work associated with a years-ago acquaintance rape.

"Her pushes were energetic, but not enough. After several hours of working and positioning, perineal floor massage and coaching I began to understand that her pushes were going only just so far. She was pushing at or to her baby, but she would not push through her pelvis.

"As I explained this to her, searching for ways to help her draw up the power she needed to succeed, her mate softly added his thoughts. He asked her if perhaps she might be holding back buried emotion as a result of her experience of violation. She quietly considered this as we all rallied our support. Although she felt she had not been deeply impacted by the brief assault she had indeed been unconsciously keeping an area of herself walled off in resistance. Now surrounded by those who loved her, the wall came down.

"She changed position and took a break. I stepped out into the forest for a moment of solitude. Throughout it all, the baby had reassured us with vibrant scalp color, responsiveness and excellent heart tones. Focused with new direction, we began again. She held nothing back and pushed like an avalanche. We soon had our baby; the room was awash in tears.

"That night, she awakened drenched in sweat. With it she told me, a heavy cloak that had enshrouded her for many years melted away. She described the change as metamorphic, she felt like a completely new person. And she loved it.

"As with many of the women I share birth with, we kept in close touch, sharing walks and picnics along life's milestones, her transformation endured, the birth being a catalyst to finding freedom and growth she'd never imagined. More than "just" a baby was born that day" (Sagaday, 1995).

For some women birth may be a physical process to be got through in order to have a baby and for others it can be part of their spiritual lives. Whatever her experience it is important that a woman should be undisturbed and given quiet encouragement whenever possible.

Pain During the Second Stage of Labour

The experience of pain in labour and birth is as much cultural as it is biological (see Oakley and Houd, 1990; Oakley, 1980) and how a woman copes with pain will be affected by this (Leap, 1996).

British culture, encouraged by medical attitudes, and an historical perception of women as weak and fragile and unable to cope (Murphy-Lawless, 1998) promotes the idea that normal childbirth is excruciatingly painful for all women.

As a result, increasing numbers of women approach childbirth in fear and trepidation based on the films and TV programmes they have seen, and tales from friends or relatives who have experienced painful, medically managed, births.

This increases the reliance on analgesia and anaesthesia and encourages the belief that caesarean section may be a preferable option to vaginal birth even when there are no complications.»

"It was still very painful and I felt very confused –
it was very hard work."

» There comes a point in most women's labours when it can be extremely painful. In a normal labour this should not be for a prolonged period, or continuous. However, when women's labours are induced or accelerated they often find that it is extremely painful for the duration of their labours and it is unusual for them not to need pharmocological pain relief (see Thomas, 1998).

Women's reactions to pain during the birth of a baby differ. For some women the second stage of labour is experienced as a relief from the contractions of the first stage of labour. For some women it can seem more purposeful or relaxed, and enjoyable. For other women this is a time of great intensity, confusion and pain.

> *"Suddenly I felt totally elated. I was excited because I knew we were getting there and I was completely in control of what was happening. Now I was having gaps between the contractions and could even tell Nic I loved him, which was wonderful. There was a great sense of opening up emotionally as well as physically."*

The reaction of midwives, doctors, and companions to the woman's pain also differs, and may affect the course of her labour and how she deals with it. The experienced midwife who knows the woman, will help support her through the process, rather than offer pharmaceutical pain relief and risk taking the experience away from her (Leap, 1996).

> *"The all-fours position was most bearable for contractions and I found my involuntary deep howling actually purged the pain from my body. Yet so often women in labour are told to keep quiet! The intensity of the second stage was the same as before – it was a repeat of that death-like state – however without artificial analgesia and with a naturalbuild up I coped easily, despite at one stage saying 'Never Again'"*
>
> (From Birth Reclaimed, Part 2,
> Green Line, No 29, Feb. 1985)

The midwife and the woman will also know if the judicious use of pain relief is needed. »

As the second stage unfolds the woman may need calm and quiet support and encouragement and genuine feedback about how the birth is progressing (Anderson, 2000), or if the woman wants by using a mirror to show her how close she is to the birth, or suggesting she puts her fingers in her vagina to feel the baby's head herself.

Very rarely, pain could be a message that all is not well. If a woman experiences continuous or overwhelming pain during a normal birth where she has been coping well, the midwife will check to see whether or not there is a problem.

The relationship between the woman and her midwife is very significant in determining how the woman will cope with and look back on her labour and birth (Simkin, 1990). Yet with few exceptions (Kirkham, 2000) this relationship is little acknowledged in most birth settings. We have thus looked briefly at the development of birth practices in the West to explore some of the thinking behind these which has led to the second stage of labour being routinely managed.

» Increasing numbers of women are using water pools for pain relief. These pools, unlike pharmacological drugs, have no side effects, and offer very effective pain relief for the majority of women who use them. If, however, it is not effective the woman can always get out and obtain other methods of pain relief. For further information on using water in labour and birth (see Further Reading – Beech, 1998).

History of Second Stage Management

The orthodox 'active' rather than 'physiological' approach to the second stage of labour has its origins in the increasing management of birth during the 18th century. This was refined around the 1920s. In many ways it remains relatively unchanged today (see Thomson, 1995; and Watson, 1994b). Little critical analysis appeared until the 1970s (Simkin, 1990) and even now it remains a relatively under-researched and debated area, though over the last few years, more discussion has appeared in midwifery and medical journals.»

As with many issues in childbirth, women's views and experiences are not well documented. A notable exception to this is researcher Josephine Green's work which suggests that women's perceptions of birth outcomes include their experiences of the second stage of labour (Green, 1998).

During the 20th century doctors became increasingly forceful in promoting what they perceived to be a "scientific" approach to every phase of the birth process (see Murphy-Lawless's compelling 1998 critique of the medicalisation of birth).

» See commentaries on the second stage of labour by Cruttenden, 1995; Downe, 1997; d'Entremont, 1996; Flint, 1997; McLean, 1995; Palmer, 1996; Sagady, 1995; Stamp, 1998; Thomson, 1995; Thomson, 1997; Watson, 1994a; Watson, 1994b.

In the early part of the 20th century the second stage in particular was seen as dangerous and in need of careful management. Many believed that the longer this stage took, the more traumatic it was for woman and baby, and the worse the outcome would be for the baby.

Some American obstetricians promoted the idea of by-passing the second stage altogether by using forceps, and episiotomy (cutting the perineum) under general anaesthetic as soon as the woman's cervix was fully dilated (De Lee, 1920; Pomeroy, 1918). Medical textbooks at that time included statements such as:

"...every minute the baby's head is on the perineum two points can be deducted from its IQ."

"The fetal brain suffers prolonged pounding and congestion in a hard spontaneous delivery with possible brain damage and anoxemia [sic] or asphyxia."

The fetal head was described as "a battering ram wherewith to shatter...a resisting outlet". The second stage was also compared to the woman falling on a pitch-fork which pierces the perineum, and the baby having its head crushed in a door.

These powerful images, along with the belief that labour should not exceed certain time limits, generated the feeling of fear and danger and the predominant belief was that the faster the second stage, and indeed labour overall, the better for both woman and baby. This unfounded belief formed one of the bases on which 'active management' of labour was subsequently developed.

Active Management of the Second Stage of Labour

"There is probably no organ that is so uncontrolled and so erratically inefficient as the human uterus. In ancient times it used to wander about the body and cause hysteria in the process. At least, that is what it was thought to do. Nowadays and thanks to medical knowledge, it is fixed to its ligaments, but this has by no means bridled its erratic behaviour. If only ancient writers had considered that uteri do not wander within bodies but among countries and continents, the term hysteria would have been more aptly derived than it is now.

The larger the uterus, the greater is the hysteria that it can inflict upon its surroundings. Thus, if a pregnant uterus wanders into France, it becomes so hyperactive that there is more than a 40-percent chance that it will need subduing by a range of tocolytic drugs in order to prevent untimely expulsion of the baby.

On the other hand, if it wanders into Ireland, it becomes so sluggish that no tocolytic agents are marketed in the country and the odds are two to three that it will need to be driven on by syntocin to expel a baby that would have fallen out a long time ago, if only it had stayed in France. If it crosses the Atlantic, the chances are that neither of these attempts to curb erratic uterine behaviour will be effective and that one uterus in five will need a scalpel to bring it to its senses and release its contents.

Surely, there is only one solution for an organ that is so erratic and so poorly controlled: 'active management'!"
(Extract of a tongue in cheek article by obstetrician Marc Keirse, 1993)

"Active management" originated in Dublin, Ireland, at the National Maternity Hospital and was developed by obstetrician Keiran O'Driscoll, primarily to manage birth – but also as a means of processing women and babies through a busy hospital labour ward as quickly as possible (O'Regan, 1998).

In Westernised countries, discussions have focused on the relative merits of "active management" of labour. During the second stage of labour this often involves the women being in a semi-reclining position, and includes care-givers instructing the woman to hold her breath and push for as long and as hard as she can from the beginning to the end of each contraction.

As midwife Ann Thomson observed, "the woman is constantly exhorted not to waste her pains and the encouragement given can make the delivery room appear to be similar to a rugby scrum" (Thomson, 1995).

Variations on active management may include any or all of the following:

No
- Encouraging women to lie down or sit propped up on a bed or a mattress.

- Speeding up labour with syntocinon if the woman's cervix does not dilate by 1cm an hour, once she is in labour.

No
- Imposing time limits regardless of the well being of woman and baby.

No
- Breaking the woman's waters (artificial rupture of membranes – ARM).

No
- Checking the dilation of the woman's cervix and the position of the baby's head by carrying out an internal vaginal examination to "assess progress" at regular intervals.

No
- Instructing the woman to push vigorously as soon as her cervix is fully dilated – often before she has any urge to bear down.

- Instructing her to tuck her chin onto her chest, take a big breath and push for as long and as hard as she can (often called the Valsalva manoeuvre, see page 59).

- If she seems a little confused initially, inserting one or more fingers into her vagina in an attempt to "teach" her where to push, rather than enabling her to find her own way of bearing down.

Active management was promoted to women as a means of "guaranteeing" that no woman would labour for longer than twelve hours (O'Driscoll and Meagher, 1993) and, by hastening the birth, allegedly making it safe.

This method focuses on "correctly" diagnosing the start of labour and from that moment it is required to conform to a strict timetable, where the woman's cervix has to dilate by 1 cm per hour. If it does not comply with this regime, the woman has her waters broken and a syntocinon drip set up. She would also, usually, be immobilised on a bed and attached to an electronic fetal monitor and as a result experienced very painful contractions.

Most large, centralised, obstetric units in the UK have adopted selected parts or variations of this regime. Interestingly, the constant presence of a midwife – which is part of active management and the only positive aspect of this form of care which can be supported by scientific evidence (Thornton, 1994) has not been adopted, and in many hospitals women are left on their own with their partners, who are often, understandably, very anxious.

As a result of lack of continuous support and reassurance, most women find the increased pain difficult to cope with and need pain relief. Epidural anaesthesia is often used, despite the possible drawbacks of increased rates of longer labours, caesareans and assisted deliveries (Thorp and Breedlove, 1996).

Research shows that the continuous presence of a known and trusted midwife is greatly valued by women who emphasise the confidence, support and reassurance that knowing one's midwife provides (McCourt and Page, 1996) and that an experienced female companion shortens the length of labour, reduces the need for pharmaceutical pain relief and reduces the intervention rates (Klaus et al, 1986; Hodnett, 2000).

Common Interventions

Vaginal examinations (VEs) No

Vaginal examinations have become a routine part of labour care, particularly to assess full dilation of the cervix to decide when to instruct the woman to push. However, clinicians have recognised that there are substantial variations in estimates of dilatation by different observers in the same situation, and even by the same observer on repeat examination (see Crowther et al, 2000; and Robson, 1992).

VEs can be painful (McKay and Barrows, 1991) particularly if women have had their labours accelerated with a prostin pessary, and researchers have suggested they can also be intimidating and ritualistic (Bergstrom et al, 1992) and more so if the midwife is unwilling to perform an examination with the woman in an upright position.

There is also the risk that a woman will not have time, or not feel able, to get up again if she is persuaded to lie down, at the beginning or during the second stage of labour. Furthermore if the midwife finds during the VE that the woman is fully dilated, this may lead to time limits being imposed on her second stage.

A woman has a right to decline any vaginal examination. In one unit in Sheffield, midwives have a policy of not carrying out VEs routinely, and will only do so if the woman and her midwife think it useful or necessary. However, many midwives may be nervous about judging the progression of labour without undertaking a VE.

Skilled midwives often rely on observing the woman's behaviour and listening to the sounds she is making rather than performing a vaginal examination at this delicate stage (Warren, 1999).

Artificial rupture of membranes (ARM)

Breaking the waters (usually referred to as ARM or amniotomy) according to Marc Keirse and Ian Chalmers (1989) "represents one of the most irrevocable interventions in pregnancy (and) constitutes obstetric interference of the most profound nature. More than any other interventions currently used to induce labour, it embodies a firm commitment to delivery."

ARM is commonly used in British hospitals as a means of inducing labour (when it is carried out before the woman is in established labour) or accelerating a woman's labour which is perceived as too slow. Once ARM is performed the woman is committed to give birth within 24 hours as this procedure introduces the possibility of infection.

"I went into hospital 4cm dilated. I had an internal examination and the midwife told me that she was going to break my waters, I protested, and she told me it was for the baby's and my own good. I asked why, the next thing I knew they had been broken" (NCT, 1989)

Not uncommonly, a woman may be unaware that during an internal examination the birth attendant may intend to rupture her membranes. Even the gentlest midwife can inadvertently rupture the membranes during a vaginal examination, which is one of the reasons why they should only be carried out when absolutely necessary and appropriate.

The effects are variable, some women find that their labours speed up and become very painful. Others become erratic or stop altogether.

"The membranes were ruptured to accelerate the labour, which it did with a vengeance. I found it very difficult to cope with the rapid increase in rate and strength of contractions" (NCT, 1989)

If the woman's labour stops the staff will seek medical assistance. If this occurs at home the woman may end up being transferred to hospital. Experienced home birth midwives consider that ARM should not be used at home because of the risks of complications developing. On rare occasions, however, where both the woman and the midwife agree that breaking the waters would assist the woman's labour to progress the judicious use of ARM can be helpful.

It is difficult to determine how often this intervention is used in childbirth as the Office of Populations Censuses and Surveys does not collect data, but one study (Moran-Ellis, 1991) revealed that 54.5% of women who responded to a survey had undergone ARM.

Lying or sitting on a bed

Women in the UK are still frequently encouraged to labour lying or sitting on a bed. As discussed earlier (see page 29), any supine position immobilises the woman and lying back propped up on pillows also causes the woman to experience greater pain and can slow down the labour and birth.

"To stand up was bearable, to sit down was painful, to lie down was excruciating."

These positions can also affect the baby's hearbeat, as it may slow down the flow of blood (and hence oxygen) to the woman's placenta. Some midwives will suggest that the woman should "just pop up on the bed now" (often in order to facilitate the use of electronic fetal monitoring) and she may then remain there and end up lying down or propped up with pillows.

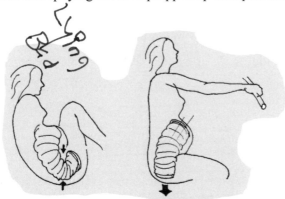

This drawing, taken from Sutton & Scott (1995), illustrates the difficult journey the baby must negotiate when the mother is propped up, compared to the relatively straightforward passage when the mother is upright.

The woman may feel more in control propped up – but physiologically this position is actually worse than lying flat, because it compresses the pelvic outlet and the pelvis is even less able to open up in the way it is designed to for birth, making the space that is available less negotiable for the baby (see Sutton and Scott, 1995).

Studies have shown that for most women lying on one's back to give birth also results in more tears and episiotomies, more forceps deliveries, more traction applied with the use of forceps, fewer spontaneous third stages and increased lower back strain (see Hoult et al, 1977; Howard, 1958; Newton and Newton, 1960; Inch, 1989).

Electronic fetal heart monitoring (EFM)

In many hospitals midwives have lost the skill of listening to baby's heartbeats and instead rely on electronic fetal monitors.» These monitors usually require the woman to lie on a bed, or sit still on a chair, while an ultrasound transducer is strapped to her abdomen to record the baby's heartbeat and the woman's contractions. There is no reason why the woman should not be in a more upright position, kneeling forward for example – but if she moves, the transducer tends to fall off.

» Many midwives now use hand held Doppler monitors, called Sonicaids. These are small unobtrusive machines using ultrasound to listen to the baby's heart beat at intervals, which some women and midwives prefer. However, there is a risk that while midwives are using these monitors they are losing the skill of listening with a Pinard stethoscope (a small ear trumpet) and observing the woman's behaviour. This method may be preferred by women who wish to avoid using a Sonicaid so as not to expose their babies to ultrasound.

There is good evidence that continuous EFM is of no value and has disadvantages for fit and healthy woman experiencing normal, physiological labours (Thacker, 1998). Some women, however, particularly if they have had a previous still birth or other tragic loss, may want EFM for reassurance.

Hospital policies nearly always include a 20 minute EFM trace on admission to hospital and constant electronic monitoring throughout labour, using a machine with a belt is still not unusual. This technology was introduced widely into clinical practice during the 1970s and 1980s in the absence of any evidence that it was either effective or safe. It is currently used on over 70% of women in labour in the UK (see Rosser, 1998).

Indeed, a systematic review of the clinical trials on EFM has shown that intrapartum electronic monitoring significantly increases the chances of caesarean operations and operative vaginal deliveries without any apparent benefits in terms of neonatal outcome (Thacker, 1999).

EFM is intrusive, and not easily interpreted, it also restricts the woman's movements and inhibits her from focusing on the challenging job of giving birth. It has also been shown to increase the pain of labour and increase the risk of operative vaginal deliveries (see Kennedy, 1998; Thacker, 1995).

While electronic fetal monitors might have a value in selected cases where the baby may be compromised, and therefore need continuous monitoring, there is no evidence that they have reduced morbidity, or perinatal or neonatal mortality rates (see Wagner, 1994).

Despite the evidence, it may be useful to know that many hospitals have a risk management policy which is based on the requirements of insurance arrangements which reward, by lower premiums, those Trusts that carry out certain procedures – such as a 20 minute monitoring trace on admission.

With the exception of sociologist Jo Garcia and colleague's early work (1985) few studies have explored women's experiences of continuous EFM, but research has reported a tendency for monitored women to be left alone (Hodnett, 2000) and for the staff and partners to take less notice of the woman when a monitor is used (Klaus, 1993).

When EFM is used, the machine rather than the woman tends to become the focus of attention. It can also have a considerable impact on the father, as related by a midwife's report of a father's story of his first son's birth and her subsequent change of practice:

"Suspected fetal distress was an ongoing concern throughout the labour with various doctors and midwives adopting a 'wait and see' approach. Little of their deliberations were communicated to the parents and the information that was given was ambiguous (as is often the case with EFM interpretations). Uncertainty persisted until, in late second stage, a forceps delivery was carried out for slow progress and suspected fetal distress. His son was born in good condition and there was relief all round but it was the father's most terrifying experience of his life. He thought his child would be born brain damaged. That story had a profound impact on the midwife and she no longer routinely applies EFM for normal labour". (Walsh, 2000).

In many cases where the EFM is showing indications that the baby is in distress the staff will suggest using a fetal scalp electrode, in the belief that this will improve the accuracy of the tracings. Fetal heart monitoring involves inserting an 'S' shaped double ended needle into the baby's scalp and, apart from the risks associated with breaking the waters, this procedure also increases the risk of infection. Donald Okada's (1977) study of infections associated with fetal scalp electrodes found an incidence of 4.5%.**»**

Fetal blood sampling

This technology was developed because of the frequent misinterpretation of EFM, as a means of double-checking whether or not the baby was in distress. This is done by taking a sample of the baby's blood by inserting a needle into its scalp.

A review of ten randomised controlled trials of EFM revealed that the use of fetal blood sampling was not associated with any benefits such as a reduction in

» A study by Linda Needs (1992) compared three different types of fetal scalp electrode and found different rates of trauma between different types of electrode. If a scalp electrode is used on your baby, insist that the type and name of the maufacturer is inserted in your medical records, as you may need to know this in future. Names of drugs used on you and your baby are recorded. It is, therefore, equally important to have records of the types of equipment used.

unnecessary caesarean sections (Thacker and Stroup, 1998; and Rosser, 1998). It concludes: "The use of fetal blood sampling (which was previously recommended as an adjunct to EFM as it was believed to reduce the number of unnecessary caesarean sections) is no longer of demonstrable benefit".

Time limits during the second stage of labour – what is usual

There is obviously a need to ensure that the woman and her baby are well during the second stage of labour. As we have already seen, during the resting phase of the second stage measurable "progress" may not occur and is not essential (see 'Rest and Be Thankful, page 18). During the active phase, as long as the woman and baby are well (Patterson et al, 1992) and there are signs of some progress, there appear to be no justifiable medical grounds for intervention (see Watson, 1994b).

However, as we have already suggested the majority of British hospitals have adopted variations of active management of labour and the imposition of time limits on labour and birth. These are based on Friedman's curve» which itself has a questionable basis (Albers et al, 1996; see Murphy Lawless, 1998). These time limits can often create a sense of urgency which interfere with the birth process and increase the use of interventions.

» Friedman's Curve is a graph which plots cervical dilatation in centimetres against time in hours. It was based on 100 primigravid women (having their first babies) in spontaneous labour in hospital. No exclusions were made, for example, for malposition, multiple pregnancy or the use of oxytocin. More importantly, it also takes no account of the individuality of women and babies and the birth process.

One researcher noted that a normal second stage may last many hours without the baby suffering ill-effects, although the longer the second stage the greater the likelihood of instrumental or operative delivery – after 5 hours in the second stage the prospects of spontaneous birth in the subsequent hour are only 10-15% (Menticoglou et al, 1995).

In their chapter on the second stage the authors of *A Guide to Effective Care in Pregnancy and Childbirthirth* conclude that "There is no evidence that a policy of early bearing down has any compensating advantages for either the mother or the baby (see Enkin et al, 2000). *Myles Textbook for Midwives* states that, "There is no good evidence to suggest that the imposition of an upper time limit for duration of the second stage improves the outcome for woman and baby" (see Sleep, 1993).

Similarly, a recent randomised controlled trial concluded that active labour in healthy women lasts longer than is widely appreciated and that a longer period of time in the second stage can be justified (Albers, 1997).

The Valsalva manoeuvre: push! push! push!

"Once I was fully dilated the midwife urged me to push. I didn't really feel any urge to do so and never really got into the rhythm of it. I feel I might have done if I'd been left for a while, until I felt like pushing."

The physiological response to the second stage has already been described (see page 26). In contrast, the active management approach involves directing women to push their babies out as quickly as possible. As already described, this 'directed pushing' requires women repeatedly to take a big breath in, hold it and push as hard as she can for as long as she can during contractions.»

APGAR Scores

Research has also found no relation between the time spent in the second stage of labour and low APGAR scores (a subjective measurement of babies well being assessed at 1 minute and 5 minutes after birth). "Second stage labours of up to 3 hours duration do not seem to carry undue risk to the fetus" (Patterson et al, 1992). Other researchers found no relation between longer second stages of labour and the frequency of low APGAR scores or the number of babies admitted to Special Care Baby Units (Saunders et al, 1992).

Research also indicates that bradycardia (a sustained fall of the baby's heartbeat) first appearing during late second stage of labour is not associated with poor APGAR scores and that there appear to be no disadvantages to a healthy baby in later life when this phase lasts up to three hours (Cohen 1977; Saunders, 1992; Menticoglou et al, 1995) or even longer.

» During exertion when performing heavy physical tasks, studies have shown that there is only a little air in the chest for maximum effort (Blankfield, 1965).

This sustained breath holding and pushing (the Valsalva manoeuvre) was originally used by a 17th century Italian doctor, who described holding the breath and straining in order to force pus out of the middle ear (see Inch, 1989). It seems likely that this was adopted by obstetrics to help women give birth quickly in unfavourable positions.

The Valsalva maneouvre has a number of potentially harmful effects on both woman and baby. In the woman it can cause sudden falls and rises in blood pressure (Caldeyro-Barcia, 1978). It can alter her heart rate patterns and brain wave patterns. Burst capillaries in the face and eyes are not uncommon and very rarely it can cause strokes (see Inch, 1989).

Early forceful pushing is ineffective and can exhaust the woman and baby. At best it may discourage the woman and those with her and, at worst, may reduce the amount of oxygen available to her and her baby and thus contribute to fetal distress (Caldeyro-Barcia 1978; see also below). Waiting until the baby has descended and the woman feels like bearing down is associated with more spontaneous births (Maresh 1983; Benyon 1990).»

There is no evidence to suggest that women need to be directed about when and how to push (see Sleep, 2000) and the practice of breath holding may indeed be harmful (Thomson, 1995).

» When pushing is undesirable or impossible, perhaps due to maternal heart problems or paralysis, often labour progresses well, reducing the use of forceps and episiotomies (Benyon, 1990). Midwives have also observed that when a woman has an epidural, often two hours are "allowed" once her cervix is fully dilated, to let the baby's head descend. If there is no epidural the tendency is to encourage early pushing.

A recent study observed that when a group of women pushed spontaneously, none of them took a deep breath before bearing down (Thomson, 1995).

Most midwives are aware of the adverse effects of directed pushing (Thompson, 1993; Yeates and Roberts, 1984) and that vigorous encouragement to push is no longer acceptable practice. But there are still wide variations in policies and practices in different hospitals and between different practitioners in Britain.

AIMS has, over recent years, received complaints from women who suffered third degree tears to the perineum during birth. Every one of them was instructed to push on command, and though many of them said that they had no pushing sensation they felt they had to follow the midwives' instructions.

The effects of directed, vigorous pushing during the second stage of labour on the woman's pelvic ligaments, muscles and tissues are not well understood or documented.

One of the clearest explanations is given in a paper reprinted in "Episiotomy and the Second Stage of Labour" (Beynon, 1990). She argues that directed pushing usually involves encouraging the woman to push from the very onset of each contraction. It appears however that the early part of the contraction draws the woman's internal structures tight and allows the vaginal muscles to be held taut, stopping the bladder supports and ligaments from being pushed down.

In her paper, Beynon describes the relationship between the woman's vaginal wall and bladder supports, the baby's head and the effect of early forceful pushing; as opposed to bearing down as and when the woman feels like it.

She uses the image of a coat sleeve with an inner lining and considers the effect of an arm being thrust down the sleeve: it is likely that the lining will roll out at the bottom. If the arm, however, is lowered carefully and slowly down the sleeve, less of the lining is likely to roll forward.

If, in addition, the lining is held firmly in place at the shoulder, it will stay in place as the arm is lowered down the sleeve. Using this analogy a less vigorous approach to the second stage may reduce the risk of the vaginal wall and bladder supports being pushed forward during birth.

She also suggests that birth attendants using forceps should take account of this and apply traction after the initial onset of the contraction which acts a bit like the lining of a sleeve being held at the shoulder.

It is thought that straining these ligaments and supports may be linked to incontinence and prolapse in later life. There is some evidence to support this theory (Malpas, 1955). Interestingly, in an observational study by midwife/researcher Ann Thomson (1995) none of the women in the spontaneous pushing group pushed at the beginning of a contraction.

Some women, surprisingly, manage to focus on their own instincts and ignore instructions urging them to push for as long and as hard as they can.»

"When the midwife said hold your breath and push, I just interpreted it in my own mind to breathe out, open and relax. As I was on all-fours facing away from her, she couldn't see what I was doing. I just breathed the baby out. It was a wonderful experience – so gentle and natural, I had no tears or problems".

The baby can also be affected by vigorous pushing. As mentioned above, the woman's lungs fill with a large volume of air, causing high enough pressure in her chest cavity to slow the flow of blood back from the heart and therefore to the placenta and the baby (Caldeyro-Barcia, 1978). The normal exchange of oxygen which takes place in the lungs is also adversely affected, so that the decreased amount of blood that reaches the baby is less oxygenated.

At the end of the first stage of labour, dips in the baby's heart rate are not uncommon but most babies recover at the onset of the second stage (see Robertson, 1988). The Valsalva manoeuvre may jeopardise this recovery and cause the very problem it is designed to prevent.

» A woman who has an effective epidural may be at increased risk of pelvic floor damage because she will be told when and how to push and will not be aware of any bodily sensations which might protect her from harm.

A study (Barnett and Humenick, 1982) found that in contrast to the women who pushed spontaneously, those babies born to women who were instructed to push experienced severe decelerations (dips in the baby's heart rate) during birth.

Roberto Caldeyro-Barcia (1978) found that when a woman finds her own rhythm to bear down, she will do so for 5-6 seconds, perhaps several times during a contraction. This caused transient drops in the babies' heart rates, followed by a quick recovery. When bearing down was prolonged, even slightly, to 9 seconds, the babies heart rates fell lower and stayed lower for longer.»

» Midwives have noticed that when a baby is being continuously monitored the harmful effects of prolonged breath holding can clearly be seen. The baby's heart rate usually recovers if the woman stops holding her breath.

Possible Complications of the Second Stage of Labour

The baby's position

The baby's position can make a difference to how the second stage of labour progresses. The ideal position for the baby during labour and birth seems to be the occipito-anterior position, where the baby's back lies towards the front of the woman's belly. If your baby is in this position prior to the birth it is possible to feel your baby's back as you run your hand down the side of your abdomen.

Jean Sutton (Sutton and Scott, 1995) asserts that women whose babies are in this position are more likely to go into spontaneous labour and have shorter and easier labours; and that babies in the left occipito-anterior (LOA) position are less likely than right occipito-anterior (ROA) babies to turn to a posterior position during labour, which can result in a longer and more difficult labour.»

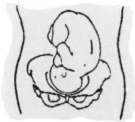

Left occipito anterior

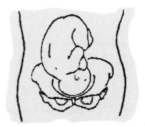

Right occipito anterior

The occipito-posterior (OP) presentation is less common and as well as causing a longer labour, may cause the woman to experience painful backache, although this is not always the case. If your baby is still posterior when you go into labour you can encourage him/her to turn by staying upright, kneeling and leaning forward and by walking around, circling your hips and changing your position as you want to. Many babies settle into the LOA position before labour or in early labour.

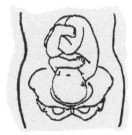
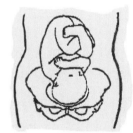

Left occipito posterior   **Right occipito posterior**

Can the second stage of labour take too long?

The second stage may take some time due to physiological, emotional, or environmental influences – or indeed a complex combination of these. Because of the influence of active management of labour and partograms

---

» Jean Sutton and Pauline Scott (1995), were so concerned about the numbers of women who were experiencing birth difficulties related to the positioning of babies, and about women sitting or lying on their backs to give birth, they published a booklet "Understanding and Teaching Optimal Foetal Positioning". You may wish to obtain a copy of the booklet and discuss their recommendations with your partner, and/or birth supporter and your midwife (see Further Reading, page 83 for details).

charts which record the progress of a labour, the baby's heart rate, the woman's contractions, blood pressure and pulse), there is a general expectation that labour will only last a specific time.

As mentioned earlier, time in itself is not a good reason to intervene if the woman and the baby are well. If there are genuine concerns based on evidence of a problem this should be fully discussed with the woman who may need help to birth her baby. Ultimately her needs and wishes should remain paramount.

The woman may feel no bearing down urge because the second stage is progressing well and it is not necessary for her to do so. However, an epidural will often delay this stage of labour as the woman has no sensation of bearing down to work with, the muscle tone of the pelvic floor is reduced, and she is often lying down on a bed. (Low-dose epidurals sometimes enable women to maintain mobility, but not always).

> *"I got quite despondent because I couldn't feel anything happening.*
> *Without feeling, it's just a concept of pushing –*
> *I had to keep thinking about it."*

Rarely the baby may be genuinely too large for the woman's pelvis or, more commonly, may be in an awkward position, but this will often be suspected before the beginning of the second stage (when this is the case changing position, particularly being more upright, standing or squatting, could help).

The woman may be exhausted from a long and challenging first stage of labour. She may have had little or nothing to eat or drink for a long time. A rest and nutritious drink or small snack at this point may give her extra strength to enable her to birth her baby.

The woman might be worried about "making a mess" as she feels pressure on her bowel, and may find it helpful to sit on the toilet or adopt a hands and knees position.

She may be fearful of so much sensation, so much stretching, or of tearing and damaging herself or her baby. Reassurance and encouragement to express her fears, and let go, can be helpful.

She may not have moved for some time and may need encouragement to do so (Roberts and Woolley, 1996). Some women need a lot of physical support to change their position at this stage, because they feel so tired and heavy. This is not such a problem for women using pools for birth because the buoyancy of the water makes any movement easier.

Occasionally, there may be deep-seated emotional reasons causing fear and panic (Gaskin, 1977). These are best dealt with antenatally, perhaps with the help of a skilled counsellor, but could be resolved at the time of birth by an intuitive attendant or friend. (See 'Emotional aspects of the second stage of labour', page 37)

Fetal distress

Some babies can become distressed for a variety of reasons during labour. However, one of the problems highlighted by research is the relatively poor ability of doctors and midwives to detect fetal distress accurately. A study at a hospital in England reinforced the view that, even where staff are well-trained, interpretation of electronic fetal heart traces cannot be relied upon (Murphy et al, 1990). Indeed, there is little known about a baby's normal heart rate in an undisturbed second stage as interpretations of electronic fetal monitoring were introduced without first establishing the range of normal heartbeats.»

Two studies showed that healthy babies can withstand a certain amount of oxygen deprivation and that blood is shunted from non-vital organs to vital organs to make best use of the oxygen available (Philippe, 1983; Jones and Greiss, 1982).

This may, of course, not be the case if the baby has already shown signs of distress earlier and some babies may be more vulnerable than others to oxygen deprivation. It is difficult to know because no research on these issues has been done on healthy babies born outside a controlled hospital environment.

» We know it is very difficult indeed for any woman in labour who is told that her baby is in distress to do anything other than agree to the advice she is being given. However, she does have the right to insist on a second opinion from a senior doctor or midwife. Experienced and competent midwives can be very effective advocates and advisers for parents in a dilemma about the best course of action if complications arise.

Most research is carried out in hospitals where women and their attendant's behaviour is significantly altered by the setting. Interestingly, zoologists recognising these subtle influences do not study "normal" animal and bird behaviour in zoos, they go out into the countryside into their natural environment.

Moving around and adopting upright positions, breathing and pushing as the woman feels like it seem to be the best way to avoid fetal distress. Where a baby needs help, we find that women are often aware of this, before anyone else.

Meconium staining

" Several studies have shown that the incidence of meconium-stained amniotic fluid increases as gestational age increases. The mere presence of meconium in a term pregnancy should not be alarming if there are no other signs of fetal distress". (Houlihan, 1994)

Meconium is the name given to the baby's first bowel movement which may be passed by the baby while it is still in the womb and can range in colour and consistency from pale green, brown, or yellow and watery, to black and tarry. It can be seen when the waters break spontaneously or are deliberately broken. Many midwives consider that if the baby is distressed breaking the waters will only increase it – so they do not recommend breaking the waters to check for meconium.

Meconium staining in the waters at any stage of labour is often regarded as a sign that the baby is in distress, especially during the second stage. This may or may not be the case and should not automatically be a cause for immediate obstetric intervention to deliver the baby. For example, meconium where the woman's pregnancy has exceeded 40 weeks is not usually a cause for concern (Houlihan, 1994). But before 40 weeks it could indicate a difficulty and may indicate the need for closer observation of the baby's condition. The appearance of meconium in liquor which has previously been clear may also be a cause for concern.

A multi-centre, international collaborative study (Wiswell, 2000) which examined the outcomes of 2094 babies born with meconium-stained liquor comparing those who had intubation and intra-tracheal suctioning» with those who did not. The researchers found that the intubation group of babies were significantly more likely to have lower APGAR scores and 51 had complications as a result of intubation. The researchers concluded that the practice of intubating and suctioning healthy infants with meconium-stained amniotic fluid has no benefit.»»

Should your baby need to be resuscitated you or your partner may wish to be with him/her during this procedure. Many hospitals are, however, uncomfortable with this, and you therefore may wish to find out beforehand what the policies are and negotiate about your wishes in the unlikely event that this should be necessary.

» *Intubation* – introducing a tube into the baby's windpipe to make a clear passage for air. *Intra-tracheal suctioning* – using a tube to suck out any debris.
»» Lesley Page's book (2000) "The New Midwifery" contains a detailed review of the significance of meconium – see references.

The resuscitaire can be brought into the birth room to the baby and this is routine practice in good hospitals. For a home birth the midwife should have prepared a surface upon which she can resuscitate the baby with oxygen and a bag and mask.

Episiotomy

"There is no evidence to support...claims that liberal use of episiotomy reduces the risk of severe perineal trauma, improves perineal healing, prevents fetal trauma, or reduces the risk of urinary stress incontinence after delivery. Episiotomy should be used only to relieve fetal or maternal distress, or to achieve adequate progress when it is the perineum that is responsible for lack of progress." (Sleep et al, 1984).

Episiotomy (a cut into the woman's perineum) carried out by the midwife to hasten the birth, was routinely used for women having their first babies and some having subsequent babies in most maternity units in Britain, from the 1970s until recently. Indeed, so common was this procedure that the AIMS' records even contain a report from a woman who had an episiotomy *after* the baby was born because the midwife was afraid of being reprimanded for failing to do one!

Up until 1925 most north American and British physicians agreed that episiotomy was a rarely needed emergency procedure. The campaign, led by one or two doctors, to promote prophylactic episiotomy (allegedly to reduce infant mortality and maternal morbidity) began in the USA in 1915 (see Graham, 1997), and was subsequently taken up in the UK. By the early 1980s the episiotomy rates varied in different maternity units from 15-100% (Kitzinger, 1981). A survey, published in 1986, revealed episiotomy rates as high as 96% in some hospitals (House et al, 1986). Since then, the rates of episiotomy have declined.

During the 1980s, consumer questioning of the need for routine episiotomy gained momentum. A study by midwife Jenny Sleep (1984) revealed that limiting the use of episiotomy to 10% of women resulted in neither an increase nor a major decrease in the problems experienced by women in the three months following birth. Other researchers investigated this procedure and gradually the use of routine episiotomy has declined.

However, for women having their first babies we believe that episiotomy rates in many hospitals are still too high. The Audit Commission's report *First Class Delivery* (1997) revealed that 27% of the women surveyed had had an episiotomy "but two-thirds felt that they had not had any say in the decision". It is unfortunate that there is still inadequate research demonstrating when an episiotomy may be beneficial.

Midwives, like doctors, vary in their use of episiotomy. Women may want to discuss this with their midwife beforehand. As few women will have any contact with the midwife before labour, they may want to request figures on interventions, including episiotomy rates from the hospital or ask their Community Health Council (in Scotland, the Health Council; and in

Northern Ireland, the Health and Social Services Council) to obtain them beforehand. A copy of an AIMS questionnaire seeking information about hospital statistics is available from the AIMS Publications Secretary (see page 82 for AIMS' address).

The Use of Birth Plans

The idea of a birth plan was originally introduced by the Association of Radical Midwives which suggested that women could ensure that the midwives understood what they wanted by writing a "Letter to the Midwife" (see Beech, 1991). With the fragmentation of services and hospitalised birth most women had no idea of who would be looking after them in labour. The letter was an attempt to let the midwife know what the women would like to happen in their labours.

While some midwives welcomed this development there were many midwives who looked upon the letter as an affront to their professional status and it was not uncommon to hear the comment "just who do these women think they are dictating to us"!

The Letter to the Midwife was later developed by Sheila Kitzinger who suggested that women should write a "Birth Plan" (see Kitzinger, 1999). Before long this was taken up by many hospitals which devised their own "birth plans". By this means, hospitals offered an illusion of choice, the 'tick box option', while ensuring that most women did not "choose" care the hospital did not wish to provide!

Maternity care differs, not only from area to area but also within a hospital. Birth plans are one way of attempting to get round the problems caused by lack of continuity of carer, and can be a very positive development affording the midwife the opportunity to understand the woman's wishes.

However, an obstetrician observed that women 'presenting with birth plans appeared to provide varying degrees of adverse reactions from both attendant medical and midwifery staff' (Jones et al, 1998). The researchers wondered whether women with birth plans might be receiving less support and encouragement throughout their labour than those without birth plans.

This research needs to be followed up but whether or not a birth plan is well received, we still believe it is useful if you can use it as an opportunity to talk over your views and plans with your birth companions and a midwife.

If you do decide to write a birth plan the following are points you may wish to consider regarding the second stage of labour:

- Having support from a midwife in establishing a gentle approach to the birth, in a calm and private environment with as little distraction as possible.

- Being given time to find your own instinctive rhythm of breathing and bearing down.
- Avoiding breath-holding and strenuous pushing (unless absolutely necessary).
- Having complete freedom of movement.
- Making any sounds that help, without inhibition or being told to be quiet.
- Eating and drinking to appetite, especially if labour is long, to avoid exhaustion and demoralisation that arise when blood sugar levels are low.
- Having encouragement from birth attendants to "open", "soften" and "let go".
- Avoiding arbitrary time limits if you and your baby are coping well.

It seems that many women and babies would benefit from adopting a more gentle approach to breathing and pushing in the second stage of labour. It could result in healthier babies, healthier women with intact perineums and undamaged internal tissues, and lead to a feeling of physical and psychological well being from which to begin the challenging and onerous task of caring for a new baby.

Labour companions

Some, all or none of the above suggestions may be of use to the woman during the birth of her baby – she will find her own ways of helping herself.

'Choosing' a Midwife

The attitude of those providing care and support for women during labour and birth is crucial to how labour progresses. A woman can choose in advance where she is going to give birth (i.e. home or hospital), but she has no choice of midwife unless she employs an independent midwife. While you do not have a right to choose a specific midwife you do have a right to refuse to be attended by anyone with whom you feel uncomfortable. The midwife or doctor has a responsibility to hand your care over to another practitioner should you exercise this right.

You may wish to consider other alternatives that enable you to get to know your carers, such as home birth or a domino birth, or, if you are fortunate, find one of the rare hospitals which offers case-load midwifery (Page, 2000) – where you will be cared for by the same midwife throughout your pregnancy and birth. However, in the light of current midwifery shortages and the medicalisation of childbirth the vast majority of hospitals do not offer case-load midwifery, or real domino births, and this is unlikely to change unless women and midwives work together to promote continuity as central to good care.

Those helping should therefore respond and be sensitive to her needs and wishes and accept, support and encourage.

During pregnancy, childbearing women, their partners, and intended labour companions may find it useful to obtain detailed information about the anatomical, physiological and emotional events of the second stage of labour, particularly the relationship between the woman's pelvis and the baby's head, and the benefits of the woman sustaining a small or medium tear rather than having an episiotomy.

It may be reassuring for them to know about the sensations of bearing down, pressure and stretching or burning and how women look, behave and sound during this stage. Information about practical ways of helping the birth of the baby progress as smoothly as possible and supporting the woman could be invaluable in increasing confidence in those helping the woman.

The woman might be helped by those attending her encouraging her to relax her jaw or to relax by massaging her buttocks and thighs, though she may not want to be touched at all. If this is her first baby, massaging the perineum during the ante-natal period and applying hot compresses during labour may be helpful (NCT, 1993; Kitzinger and Simkin, 1990).

Encouraging the woman to feel the baby's head as it crowns, perhaps even using a mirror to show her how much progress she is making may be useful. Her labour companion could use appropriate language suggesting imagining the baby's head moving through her pelvis with such words as "open, let go, soften" etc. Perhaps the companion's most valuable role is to protect the woman from outside distractions and interferences, maintaining calm and quiet support, keeping her cool and wiping her face and neck with cool or iced water, and giving her sips of water or fruit juice as desired.

Women who have had more than one birth – for instance, one where they felt unsupported and intimidated and another where they felt nurtured and encouraged – are often amazed at the differences between these experiences:

"Two and a quarter years ago, I gave birth to my first child in a large teaching hospital. After having my waters broken at 7cm, I dilated fully. However, I did not feel any urge to push. I felt confused and indecisive. The midwife's constant questioning and cajoling irritated me. She told me my baby was distressed and persuaded me to do as she suggested – lie down, push and breathe at her direction. I pushed vigorously but aimlessly, for what seemed like a long time. Lewis was born after a 17 hour labour, showing no signs of distress. I was exhausted, very swollen and had sustained a small tear. I felt confused by my body's apparent lack of direction during second stage and felt bullied by the midwife.

"Six weeks ago, I gave birth to my second son at home. I felt like laughing loudly when my waters broke, followed by a strong urge to push. I was elated. It was like someone lighting a candle in a darkened room, as I recognised what I'd read and heard about from so many women. My body was in no doubt about what to do. I felt its power and mine to help it. I yelled joyfully as Jamie entered the world, weighing 9lb 11 oz. He was born in under five hours without drugs, interventions or stitches. I was surrounded by so much loving support that the midwife's rather insensitive approach didn't bother me too much. I felt clear and active throughout my second stage. I did as I intended – resisted any interventions, squatted and breathed as I wanted, supported by friends. It was magic!" (Tracey Black, 1992)

Childbirth is perhaps one of the most overwhelming experiences in a woman's life. As she makes the final part of the journey towards seeing her baby for the first time and feels the sensations of her body, she may experience a whole range of emotions. Most women experience the moment of giving birth to their babies as awesome, almost incomprehensible perhaps. Whilst some women, for a variety of reasons may feel exhausted, numb, or disinterested and need time and support from all those around them, most women find meeting their baby for the first time a joyous and momentous occasion. These feelings and many others can be normal reactions to this challenging rite of passage.

Nadine Pilley Edwards
Beverley A Lawrence Beech
March, 2001

Further Reading

AIMS (1995) *Episiotomy – Female Genital Mutilation*, AIMS Journal, 7(2): 1-5.

Beech, BAL (ed) (1996) Waterbirth Unplugged, Books for Midiwves

Beech, BAL (1998) *Choosing a Water Birth*, AIMS

Edwards, NP (1999) *Delivering Your Placenta – The Third Stage*, AIMS.

Graham, I (1997) *Episiotomy: Challenging obstetric interventions*, Blackwell Science.

Inch, S (1989) *Birthrights*, Greenprint.

Kitzinger, S and Simkin, P (1990) *Episiotomy and The Second Stage of Labor*, Pennypress

Limburg, A and Smulders, B (1992) *Women Giving Birth*, Celestial Arts

Robertson, A (1994) *Empowering Women Teaching Active Birth in the 90's*, ACE Graphics

Robertson, A (1988) *Teaching Active Birth*, ACE Graphics

National Childbirth Trust (1993) *The Perineum in Childbirth*, Available from NCT Maternity Sales Ltd., Burnfield Ave, Glasgow, G46 7TL

Sutton, J and Scott, P (1996) *Understanding and Teaching Optimal Foetal Positioning* , Available from 7 Benedict Drive, Bedfont, Feltham, Middlesex.

Wagner, M (1994) *Pursuing the Birth Machine: The search for appropriate technology*, ACE Graphics

Thomas, P (1996) *Every Woman's BirthRights*, Thorsons

More Information

AIMS
5 Porthall Road, Brighton, BN1 5PD; Tel: 01753 652781 or 01273 506261
Web: www.aims.org.uk

For a free copy of AIMS current Publications List send an s.a.e.to:
Publications Secretary, 2 Bacon Lane, Hayling Island, Hants, PO11 ODN

ARM (Association of Radical Midwives)
62 Greetby Hill, Ormskirk, Lancs, L39 2DT; Tel: 01243 671673
Web: www.midwifery.org.uk

IMA, (Independent Midwives Association),
c/o 1 Great Quarry, Guildford, Surrey, GU1 3XN; Tel: 01483 821104
Web: www.netcomuk.co.uk/~pvan/ima.html

MIDIRS (Midwives Information and Resource Service)
9 Elmdale Road, Clifton, Bristol BS8 1SL; Tel: 01272 251 791
Web: www.midirs.org

NCT (National Childbirth Trust)
Alexander House, Oldham Terrace, London W3 6NH; Tel: 020 8992 8637
Web: www.nct-online.org

RCM (Royal College of Midwives),
15 Mansfield Street, London W1M OBE; Tel: 020 7312 3535

References

AIMS (1998) *Breech Presentation: Caesarean operation versus normal birth*, AIMS Quarterly Journal, 10(3): 1-4

Albers LL, Schiff M, Gorwoda JG (1997) *The length of active labor in normal pregnancies*, Obstetrics and Gynecology, 87(3): 355-359

Anderson T (1997) *Women's experiences of the second stage of labour.* Unpublished MSc dissertation, University of Surrey

Anderson T (2000) *Feeling safe enough to let go: The relationship between a woman and her midwife during the second stage of labour,* In: The midwife-mother relationship, Kirkham M (ed), Macmillan Press, London; p 92-118

Armstrong P, Feldman S (1987) *The Gentle Art*, Corgi

Audit Commission (1997) *First Class Delivery: Improving Maternity Services in England and Wales*, Audit Commission

Balaskas J (1991) *The New Active Birth*, Thorsons

Banks M (1998) *Breech Birth Woman-Wise*, Birthspirit Books, Hamilton, New Zealand

Barnett M and Humenick S (1982) *Infant outcome in relation to second stage labour pushing method*, Birth, 9(4): 221-229

Beech BAL (1991) *Who's Having Your Baby?,* Bedford Square Press (2nd Ed), London.

Bergstrom L, Roberts J, Skillman L and Seidel J (1992) *You'll feel me touching you, sweetie: Vaginal examinations during the second stage of labor*, Birth, 19(1): 10-18

Beynon CL (1957) *The normal second stage of labour: A plea for reform in its conduct*; Journal of Obstetrics and Gynaecology of the British Commonwealth, 64 (6)

Beynon CL (1990) *The normal second stage of labour: a plea for reform in its conduct.* In: Kitzinger S, Simkin P (eds), *Episiotomy and the second stage of labour*, Pennypress, Seattle, Washington; 23-32

Black, T (1992), personal communication

Blankfield A (1965) *The optimum positions for childbirth*, The Medical Journal of Australia; 666-668.

Caldeyro-Barcia R (1978) *Influence of maternal bearing down efforts during second stage on fetal well being*, Kaleidoscope of Childbearing: Preparation Birth and Nurturing, Pennypress.

Caldeyro-Barcia R (1985) World Health Organisation Interregional Conference on Appropriate Technology for Birth, Fortaleza, Brazil

Coates, T (1997) *Obstetric emergencies and operative procedures.* In: *Mayes Midwifery: A Textbook for Midwives*, Sweet BR and Tarin D (eds), 12th Ed., Bailliere Tindall, London; 663-668

Cohen WR (1977) *Influence of the duration of second stage labor on perinatal outcome and puerperal morbidity*, Obstetrics and Gynecology, 49 (3): 266-269

Cronk M (1998a) *Hands off the breech*, The Practising Midwife, Vol 1, No 6, p13-15

Cronk M (1998b) *Midwives and breech births*, The Practising Midwife, 1(7/8): 44-45

Cronk M (2000) *Home birth – continuity of care*, MIDIRS Midwifery Digest, 10(3): 381-382

Crowther C, Enkin M, Keirse MJNC et al. (2000) *Monitoring the progress of labour,* In: *A guide to effective care in pregnancy and childbirth,* Enkin M, Keirse MJNC, Neilson J et al. (eds), Third Edition, Oxford University Press, UK, Chapter 31; 284

Cruttenden J (1995) *To push or not to push?* Modern Midwife, 5(12): 31-32

d'Entremont M (1996) *Directed pushing in the second stage of labour,* Modern Midwife, 6(6): 12-16

de Jong PR, Johanson RB, Baxen P et al (1997) *Randomised trial comparing the upright and supine positions for the second stage of labour,* British Journal of Obstetrics and Gynaecology, 104(5): 567-571

DeLee JB (1920) *The prophylactic forceps operation,* American Journal of Obstetrics and Gynaecology, 1: 24-44

Donnison J (1988) Midwives and Medical Men: A history of the struggle for the control of childbirth, Historical Publications, London

Down S (1997) *The concept of normality in the maternity services.* In: Frith L (Ed) Ethics and the Midwife – Issues in contemporary practice, Butterworth Heinemann

Edwards NP (2000) *Women planning home birth: Their own views on their relationships with midwives.* In: The midwife-mother relationship, Kirkham M (ed), Macmillan Press; 55-91

Enkin M, Keirse MJNC, Nielson J et al (2000) *A guide to effective care in pregnancy and childbirth,* Third Edition, Oxford University Press

Evans J (1997) *Can a twin birth be a positive experience?* Midwifery Matters, 74: 6-11

Flint C (1997) *Using the stairs,* MIDIRS Midwifery Digest, 7(2): 186-187

Garcia J, Corry M, MacDonald D et al (1985) *Mothers' views of continuous electronic fetal monitoring and intermittent auscultation : a randomised controlled trial*, Birth, 12(2): 79-86

Gaskin IM (1977) *Spiritual Midwifery*, The Book Publishing Company, Summertown, USA

Graham ID (1997) Episiotomy: Challenging obstetric interventions, Blackwell Science, Oxford

Green JM, Coupland VA and Kitzinger JV (1998) *Great expectations: a prospective study of women's expectations and experiences of childbirth*, Books for Midwives Press

Gupta JK and Nikodem VC (2000) *Woman's position during the second stage of labour* (Cochrane Review). In: The Cochrane Library, Issue 2, Oxford: Update Software

Hannington-Kiff J G (1993) *Overview of obstetric epidural blocks*, AVMA Medical and Legal Journal; 2-6

Hodnett ED (2000) *Caregiver support for women during childbirth,* The Cochrane Database of Systematic Reviews, the Cochrane Collaboration Update Software 2000

Houlihan CH and Knuppel RA (1994) *Meconium-stained amniotic fluid,* Journal of Reproductive Medicine, 39(11): 888-898

Hoult IJ, MacLennan AH, Carrie LES (1977) *Lumbar epidural analgesia in labour: relation to fetal malposition and instrumental delivery*, British Medical Journal (1): 14-16

House MJ, Cario G, and Jones MH (1986) *Episiotomy and the perineum: a random controlled trial,* Journal of Obstetrics and Gynaecology, 7: 107-110

Howard FH (1958) *Delivery in the physiologic position,* Obstetrics and Gynaecology, 11(3): 318-322

Hunt S and Symonds A (1995) *The social meaning of midwifery*, Macmillan

Inch S (1989) *Birthrights*, Greenprint

Jones CM and Greiss FC (1982) *The effect of labor on maternal and fetal circulating catecholomines*, American Journal of Obstetrics and Gynecology, 144(2): 149-153

Jones MH, Barik S, Mangune H et al (1998) *Do birth plans adversely affect the outcome of labour?* British Journal of Midwifery, 6(1): 38-41

Kaufman KJ (1993) *Effective control or effective care*, Roundtable debate: active management part 2, Birth, 20(3): 150-61

Keirse MJNC and Chalmers I (1989) *Methods for inducing labour* In: Effective Care in Pregnancy and Childbirth, Chalmers I, Enkin M and Keirse RJNC (eds), First Edition, Oxford University Press; 1058

Keirse MJNC (1993) *A final comment. Managing the uterus, the woman, or whom?* Birth 20:3 p159-161

Kennedy RG (1998) *Electronic fetal heart rate monitoring: retrospective reflections on a twentieth-century technology*, Journal of the Royal Society of Medicine, 91: 244-250

Kirkham M Ed (2000) *The midwife-mother relationship*, Macmillan Press

Kitzinger S (1979) *The good birth guide*, Fontana

Kitzinger S (1985) *Women's experience of sex*, Penguin

Kitzinger S (1987) *The experience of childbirth* (6th Ed), Penguin

Kitzinger S (1999) *Birth plans: how are they being used?* British Journal of Midwifery, 7(5): 300-303

Kitzinger S, Simkin P (1990) *Episiotomy and the second stage of labour*, Pennypress

Kitzinger S, Walters R (1981) *Some women's experiences of episiotomy*, National Childbirth Trust; 1

Klaus MH, Kennell JH, Klaus PH (1993) *Mothering the mother: how a doula can help you have a shorter, easier and healthier birth*, New York: Addison Wesley

Klaus MH, Kennel JH, Robertson SS, Sosa R (1986) *Effects of social support during parturition on maternal and infant morbidity*, British Medical Journal, 293: 585-587

Leap N (1996) *A midwifery perspective on pain in labour*. Unpublished Master's Dissertation, South Bank University, London

Malpas P (1955) Genital prolapse and allied conditions, Barvey and Blythe

Maresh M, Choong KH and Beard RW (1983) *Delayed pushing with lumbar epidural analgesia in labour*, British Journal of Obstetrics and Gynaecology, 90: 623-627

McCandlish R (1997) *Care during the second stage of labour*. In: Alexander J, Levy V, Roth C (eds) Midwifery Practice: Care Topics 2, MacMillan Press Ltd; 98-112

McCandlish, R, Bowler, U, van Astin, H (1998) *A randomised controlled trial of care of the perineum during second stage of normal labour*, British Journal of Obstetrics and Gynaecology, 105(12): 1262-1272

McCourt C, Page L (1996) *Report on the evaluation of one-to-one midwifery*, Thames Valley University, London

McKay S, Barrows T (1991) *Holding back: maternal readiness to give birth*, American Journal of Maternal and Child Nursing, 16(5): 250-254

McLean MT (1995) *The medicalization of the second stage of labor*, Midwifery Today; 33: 36

Mendez-Bauer C et al (1976) *Effects of different maternal positions during labour*, 5th European Congress on Perinatal Medicine, Sweden

Menticoglou SM, Manning F, Harman C and Morrison I (1995). *Perinatal outcome in relation to second-stage duration*, American Journal of Obstetrics. and Gynecology; 173(3 Part 1): 906-912

Moran-Ellis J (1991) *Rupture of membranes in labour*, Journal of Obstetrics and Gynaecology; 11(Supl 1): S6-S10

Morrin NA (1997) *Midwifery care in the second stage of labour*, In Mayes' Midwifery – A Textbook for Midwives, Ed Sweet BR, Tarin D (eds), 12th Ed., Bailliere Tindall, London; 385-402

Murphy KW, Johnson J, Moorcraft J, et al (1990) *Birth asphyxia and the intrapartum cardiotocograph,* British Journal of Obstetrics and Gynaecology, 97: 470-479

Murphy-Lawless J (1998) *Reading birth and death: a history of obstetric thinking*, Cork University Press

Nakai Y, Mine M, Nishio J, et al (1998) *Effects of maternal prone position on the umbilical arterial flow*, Acta Obstetricia et Gynecologica Scandinavica, 77: 967-969

National Childbirth Trust (1989) *Rupture of the membranes in labour. A survey conducted by the National Childbirth* Turst, London

National Childbirth Trust (1993) *The perineum in childbirth: A survey conducted by The National Childbirth Trust*, London

Needs L, Grant A, Sleep J et al (1992) *A randomized controlled trial to compare three types of fetal scalp electrode.* British Journal of Obstetrics and Gynaecology, 99: 302-306

Nelson NM, Enkin MW, Saigal S, et al (1980) *A randomized clinical trial of the Leboyer approach to childbirth*, New England Journal of Medicine, 302: 324-326

Newton M, Newton N (1960) *The propped position for the second stage of labour,* Obstetrics and Gynaecology, 15(1): 28-34

Oakley A (1980) *Women confined: Towards a sociology of childbirth,* Martin Robertson, Oxford

Oakley A, Houd S (1990) *Helpers in childbirth:* Midwifery Today, Hemisphere Publications Corporation

Odent M (1998) *Physiological birth is normal birth,* Midwifery Today Conference 'Keeping Birth Normal', London Sept 10-14

O'Driscoll K, Meagher D (1993) *Active management of labour,* Third Edition, Mosby Yearbooks Europe Ltd

Okada D et al (1977) *Neonatal scalp abscess and fetal monitoring: factors associated with infection,* American Journal of Obstetrics and Gynecology, 120: 185-189

O'Regan M (1998) *Active management of labour – The Irish way of birth,* AIMS Quarterly Journal; 10(2): 1-8

Page L (2000) *The New Midwifery: Science and sensitivity in practice,* Churchill Livingstone, London

Paine LL, Tinker DD (1992) *The effect of maternal bearing-down efforts on arterial umbilical cord pH and length of the second stage of labour.* Journal of Nurse-Midwifery; 37(1): 61-63

Palmer J (1996) *Physiological pushing in the second stage of labour: the future for midwifery care,* Australian College of Midwives Incorporated Journal; 9(3): 15-19

Patterson CM, Saunders NSG and Wadsworth J (1992) *The characteristics of the second stage of labour in 25,069 singleton deliveries in the North West Thames Health Region,* British Journal of Obstetrics and Gynaecology, 99(5): 377-380

Phillippe M (1983) *Fetal catecholomines,* American Journal of Obstetrics and Gynecology; 146(7): 840-855

Pomeroy RH (1918) *Shall we cut and reconstruct the perineum for every primipara?,* American Journal of Obstetric Diseases of Women and Children

Roberts J and Woolley D (1996) *A second look at the second stage of labor,* Journal of Obstetrics, Gynaecologic and Neonatal Nursing; 25(5): 415-423

Robertson A (1988) *Teaching active birth,* Ace Graphics

Robertson A (1994) *Empowering women, Teaching active birth in the 90's,* Ace Graphics

Robson SEE (1992) *Variation of cervical dilatation estimation by midwives, doctors, student midwives and medical students in 1985 – a small study using cervical simulation models.* In: *Research and the Midwife Conference Proceedings,* 1991, University of Manchester; 26-33

Rosser J (1998) *Continuous electonic fetal heart monitoring during labour,* The Practising Midwife; 1(7/8): 60-61

Russell JGB (1982) *The rationale of primitive delivery postions,* British Journal Obstetrics and Gynaecology; 89: 712-715

Sagaday M (1995) *Renewing our faith in second stage,* Midwifery Today; 33: p29-31, 41-43

Saunders N St. G, Paterson CM and Wadsworth J (1992) *Neonatal and maternal morbidity in relation to the length of the second stage of labour,* British Journal of Obstetrics and Gynaecology; 99: 381-385

Sforza-Brewer G, Greene JP (1981) *Right from the start – meeting the challenge of mothering your unborn and newborn baby,* Rodale Press.

Simkin P (1990) *Active and physiologic management of second stage: A Review and Hypothesis*, In: Episiotomy and the second stage of labour, Kitzinger S and Simkin P, Pennypress

Sleep J (1993) *Physiology and management of the second stage of labour* In: Myles Midwifery Textbook, Bennett VR, Brown LK (eds), 12th Edition, Churchill Livingstone; 199-215

Sleep J, Grant A, Garcia J et al (1984) *West Berkshire perineal management trial.* British Medical Journal; 289: 587-590

Sleep J, Roberts J, Chalmers 1 (2000) *The second stage of labor,* In: *A guide to effective care in pregnancy and childbirth*, Enkin M, Keirse MJNC, Neilson J et al (eds), Third Edition, Oxford University Press, UK, Chapter 32: 297

Stamp G (1998) *Second stage: midwives' views and practices*, Practising Midwife; 1(6): 28-30

Sutton J, Scott P (1995) *Understanding and teaching optimal foetal positioning*, Birth Concepts, New Zealand, available from 7 Benedict Drive, Bedfont, Feltham, Middlesex

Thacker SB, Stroup DF, Peterson HB (1995) *Routine intrapartum electronic fetal monitoring decreases neonatal seizures but increases operative deliveries*, Obstetrics and Gynecology; 86: 613-620

Thacker SB, Stroup DF (1998) *Continuous electronic fetal heart monitoring during labour* (Cochrane Review) In: The Cochrane Library, Issue 2, Oxford: Update Sortware

Thacker SB, Stroup DF (1999) *Continuous electronic fetal heart monitoring during labour* (Cochrane review) In: The Cochrane Library, Issue 4, Oxford: Update Software

Thomas P (1998) *Is labour just a pain?* AIMS Journal, 10(1): 1-4

Thomson AM (1995) *Maternal behaviour during spontaneous and directed pushing in the second stage of labour*, Journal of Advance Nursing; 22: 1027-1034

Thompson T (1997) *The second stage of labour: whose urge to push?* New Zealand College of Midwives Journal; 16: 25-26

Thornton JG, Lilford R (1994) *Active management of labour – Current knowledge v research issues*, British Medical Journal; 309: 366-369

Thorp JA, Breedlove G (1996) *Epidural analgesia in labour: An evaluation of risks and benefits*, Birth; 23: 63-83

Wagner M (1994) *Pursuing the birth machine: the search for appropriate birth technology*, Ace Graphics

Walsh D (2000) *Part four: fetal monitoring should be controlled*, British Journal of Midwifery; 8(8): 511-516

Warren C (1999) *Invaders of privacy*, Midwifery Matters, 81: 8-9

Watson V (1994a) *The duration of the second stage of labour*, Modern Midwife; 4(6): 21-24

Watson V (1994b) *Maternal position in the second stage of labour*, Modern Midwife; 4(7): 21-24

Wiswell T E et al (2000) *Delivery room management of the apparently vigorous meconium-stained neonate: Results of the multi-center, international collaborative trial*, Pediatrics; 105: 1-7

Yeates DA and Roberts JE (1984) A comparison of two bearing-down techniques during the second stage of labor, Journal of Nurse-Midwifery; 29(1): 3-11